IMMIGRATION AND IDENTITY

Turmoil, Treatment, and Transformation

Salman Akhtar, M.D.

JASON ARONSON INC.
Northvale, New Jersey
London

This book was set in 11 pt. Baskerville by Alpha Graphics of Pittsfield NH
and printed and bound by Book-mart Press, Inc. of North Bergen, NJ.

Library of Congress Cataloging-in-Publication Data

Akhtar, Salman, 1946 July 31–
    Immigration and identity : turmoil, treatment, and trans-
formation / Salman Akhtar.
        p. cm.
    Includes bibliographical references and index.
    ISBN 0-7657-0232-0
    1. Emigration and immigration—Psychological aspects.
    2. Immigrants—Psychology.   I. Title.
    JV6013.A39 1999
    305.9'0691—dc21   99-28892

Printed in the United States of America on acid-free paper. For information and
catalog write to Jason Aronson Inc., 230 Livingston Street, Northvale, NJ 07647-1726,
or visit our website: www.aronson.com

To

Kabir and Nishat

arrows, shot in the bosom of the future
buds, ready to blossom in the garden of tomorrow

CONTENTS

Factors Affecting the Outcome
Circumstances of and Reasons for Migration • Access to Re-
fueling • Age at Migration • Pre-immigration Character
• Nature of the Country Left • Magnitude of Cultural Differ-
ences • Reception by the Host Population • Experiences of
Efficacy in the New Country • Birth of Children
Some Unaddressed Realms
The Role of Bodily Characteristics • The Impact of Gender •
Marriage and Immigration • Legal Status • Homosexuality
and Immigration • Dreams • The Changed Man–Animal
Relationship
Summary

PART II   IDENTITY

PART III   CROSS-CULTURAL TREATMENT

masking and Interpreting the Cultural Rationalizations of Intrapsychic Conflicts and Transference Reactions • Validating Feelings of Dislocation and Facilitating Mourning • Interpreting Defensive Functions of Nostalgia as well as Defenses against the Emergence of Nostalgia • Accepting Seemingly Inoptimal Individuation and Involvement of Relatives in Treatment • Facing the Challenge Posed by the Patient's Polyglottism and Polylingualism
Summary

PREFACE

Born in British Imperial India in 1946 and raised in that subsequently partitioned but independent and fiercely nonaligned nation, I arrived in the United States in 1973. In the twenty-six years that have followed, a panorama of transformations and triumphs has unfolded in both the academic and personal spheres of my development. One major aspect of all this has been a slow but unmistakable change in my identity, a change that is largely (though not entirely) due to my immigration.

This personal dimension is, however, not the only source of my interest in the topic of immigration. Over the last quarter of a century, I have intermingled with a large number of fellow immigrants from India and collected ethnographic bits and pieces about their lives in the context of immigration. I also have also kept in contact with ten immigrant physicians who entered the United States at about the same time I did and with whom I completed my first year of residency in psychiatry—Drs. Getulio Tovar (Brazil), Aarno Vuotila (Finland), Ravi Baliga, Harish Malhotra, Maya Malhotra, Kanan Patrawala, and Lila Rao (India), Mahmoud Malayeri (Iran), Danilo Campos (Philippines), and Young Ho Kim (South Korea). Not only did these contacts afford me an opportunity to share and observe our psychosocial growth as immigrants, they also permitted me a glimpse of the arrival and evolution of the U.S.-born off-spring of this entire group.

My interest in immigration was enhanced by studying Grinberg and Grinberg's (1989) pioneering monograph on this topic, Ticho's (1971) early paper on the cultural aspects of transference and countertransference, Garza-Guerrero's (1974) sophisticated essay on culture shock, and Amati-Mehler and colleagues' (1993) profoundly significant contribution to the issue of polylingualism and polyglottism. Reading poetry and fiction by immigrant authors of various nationalities also facilitated my understanding of the subtle and poignant issues in this realm. Contact with immigrant medical students, psychiatry residents, psychology interns, and psychoanalytic candidates of various nationalities furthered my desire to address the subject.

Yet another impetus came from undergoing psychoanalysis as an immigrant analysand whose mother tongue differed from that of his analyst, and from conducting psychotherapy and psycho-analysis with patients whose mother tongue differed from mine. This made me aware of the profound significance (and, paradoxi-cally, also of the insignificance) of linguistic difference within the therapeutic dyad. I also began to appreciate the clinical importance of difference in other idioms of personal expression (e.g., wit, optimal distance, candor, dependence, regression).

Acting in unison, such personal, social, academic, and clinical motivations led me to write a series of papers pertaining to what I was observing. My topics, at first, remained centered upon split-ting, identity, and identity diffusion (Akhtar 1984, 1992b, Akhtar and Byrne 1983, Akhtar and Samuel 1996) and only gradually started to involve the specific issues of cultural difference, immi-gration, and exile (Akhtar 1988, 1995a, 1997, 1999a,b,c). The ob-servations I made, however, remained scattered and split apart, as it were, from each other. Striving toward synthesis, I decided to weave all this material together while adding other ideas that I had not yet put down on paper. The result is this book.

It consists of three parts. Part I is entitled "Immigration" and is comprised of a single but long chapter entitled "Psychosocial Vari-ables Associated with Immigration." I begin this chapter by noting that, even under the best circumstances, immigration is a traumatic occurrence; like other traumas, it mobilizes a mourning process. I then discuss various factors that affect the psychological outcome of immigration. Among such variables, I include (1) circumstances and reasons for migration, (2) access to refueling, (3) age at migration, (4) pre-immigration character, (5) nature of the country left, (6) magnitude of cultural differences, (7) reception by the host population, (8) experiences of efficacy in the new country, and (9) birth of children in the new land. Following this, I address certain other aspects of immigration that have not received adequate (or any!) attention in the literature. These include (1) the role of bodily characteristics, (2) the impact of gender, (3) marriage and immigration, (4) legal status, (5) homosexuality and migration, (6) dreams, and (7) the changed man–animal relationship as a result of immigration.

Part II of the book is titled "Identity" and includes two chapters. Chapter 2 deals with the developmental and phenomenological aspects of identity. Here, I trace the concept of identity from its first appearance in the psychoanalytic literature in 1919 through the pertinent writings of Erikson, Lichtenstein, Jacobson, and Mahler to the contemporary revival of interest in identity-related matters. I see this revival as an antecedent to Kernberg's profound contributions to the area of severe character pathology as well as of the increasing application of psychoanalytic treatments to individuals of culturally diverse backgrounds. I discuss the various phases of identity development including the period before birth, the separation-individuation phase, Oedipus complex, latency, and adolescence. I also append a section each on the father's role in the consolidation of his children's identity, and on the refinements of identity in adulthood. Following this, I delineate seven facets of identity (realistic body image, consistent attitudes and behaviors, subjective self-sameness, temporal continuity, authenticity, gender, ethnicity and conscience) and discuss their clinical assessment and relevance. While I frequently interject comments regarding immigration in this chapter, it is in the next chapter that I bring the topics of immigration and identity together in a meaningful and deeper way.

Chapter 3 is titled "Four Tracks in Identity Transformation Following Immigration." These tracks involve the dimensions of drives and affects, interpersonal and psychic space, temporality, and social affiliation. In highlighting the immigrant's mourning–liberation process along these four dimensions, I address the issues of idealization and devaluation, closeness and distance, hope and nostalgia, the transitional area of the mind, alteration of the superego's cultural character, mutuality, and linguistic transformation. Acknowledging that the four dynamic progressions might be neither exhaustive nor independent of each other, I offer caveats to my own conceptualizations in this regard and also comment upon the more problematic situation of deeply traumatized exiles and refugees.

The ideas developed in the first two parts of the book find their relevance to our day-to-day clinical work in Part III. This part is titled "Cross-Cultural Treatment" and consists of two chapters. In Chapter 4, I offer detailed guidelines for conducting psychotherapy and psychoanalysis with immigrant patients. Not recommended as mandatory strategies, these guidelines are meant only to form a background against which the usual affirmative and interpretive interventions of deep psychotherapy or psychoanalysis should take place. These guidelines include (1) maintaining cultural neutrality and avoiding countertransference pitfalls, (2) judiciously accommodating the therapeutic framework to cultural differences, (3) adopting a developmental stance and conducting developmental work, (4) unmasking and interpreting the cultural rationalizations of intrapsychic conflicts and transference reactions, (5) validating feelings of dislocation and facilitating mourning, (6) interpreting defensive functions of nostalgia as well as defenses against the emergence of nostalgia, (7) accepting seemingly inoptimal individuation and the involvement of relatives in treatment, and (8) facing the challenges posed by the linguistic differences within the therapeutic dyad. In Chapter 5, I comment upon child and family interventions, the latter being of inestimable importance not only in the treatment of immigrant children but occasionally even in the treatment of immigrant adults, especially if they come from allocentric and collectivist cultures. I also devote a brief section each to what I term "psychoanalytically informed advice" and to the importance of community outreach programs. Following this, I address the specific dilemmas of the immigrant therapist, including his linguistic difference with his patients, his ability to maintain cultural neutrality, and his capacity to retain optimal distance between his own hybrid identity and his native patient's relatively "monoethnic" core self-representation as the two come together in the transference–countertransference crucible.

In painting the canvas of identity problems of immigrants, my palette has not been restricted to the colors of psychiatry and psychoanalysis. I have relied on my personal experience and have drawn freely from anthropology, sociology, fiction, cinema, and, above all, poetry. In doing so, I have followed my intellectual and aesthetic bent and also listened to Freud's advice. Sixty-six years ago, he ended one of his lectures by telling the audience that if they wanted to learn more about such matters they should inquire from their "own experiences of life, or turn to the poets" (Freud 1933, p. 135). I have done both!

ACKNOWLEDGMENTS

Drs. Otto Kernberg and Vamık Volkan, two immigrant psycho-analysts of international renown, have been a great source of inspiration to me. Both have contributed immensely to my personal and professional growth and I wish to express my gratitude to them here. Dr. David Hawkins, Chairman of the Department of Psychiatry at the University of Virginia School of Medicine (1967–1977), helped me obtain permanent residence in this country and I owe special thanks to him. I am also grateful to Dr. Dorothy Holmes, who arranged for me to deliver a keynote address at the Division 39 Spring Meeting of the American Psychological Association in April 1994 and suggested that I take up immigration as my topic. The talk I gave there led to my first published paper on immigration.

Next I wish to thank two individuals whose contributions to my personal and professional career, while different from each other, have indeed been profound: Raj Akhtar, with whom I migrated from India and learned the social alphabet of our new country, and with whom I have two most wonderful children, and Selma Kramer, who taught me about psychoanalysis and about life in general, in ways that were both affective and intellectual.

Formal or informal conversations with a number of immigrant colleagues within the mental health profession have also greatly benefited me. These individuals are Drs. Nora Kramer (Argentina), Anni Bergman, John Kafka, and Eric Lager (Austria), Henri Parens (Belgium), James Hamilton and Stephen Shanfield (Canada), Jun Cai (China), Mladan Stivic (Croatia), Axel Hoffer (Czechoslovakia), Hanan Hassenein, Afaf Mahfouz, and Nadia Ramzy (Egypt), Wilfred Abse (England), Maurice Apprey (Ghana), Ashwin Patkar, Dilip Ramchandani, Dwarkanath Rao, Satish Reddy, and Jagdish Teja (India), Hossein Etezady, Roknedin Safavi, and Shahrzad Siassi (Iran), Shimon Waldfogel (Israel), James Youakim (Jordan), Stuart Twemlow (New Zealand), Aisha Abbasi, Ansar Haroun, Imran Hashmi, Nasir Ilahi, and Mimi Ismi (Pakistan), John Buckman and Ruth Lax (Poland), Rita Rogers (Romania), Sabina Fila and David Nichols (Switzerland), Serra Muderrisoglu (Turkey), and Dragan Svrakic (Yugoslavia).

My dialogue with immigrant friends in Canada (Drs. Lilka Croyden, Pnina Pinchevsky, Josephine Quallenberg, and Vallabhaneni Madhusudana Rao) and England (Mr. Parvez Alam, Mrs. Sadie Gillespie, Mrs. Baljeet Mehra, Ms. Achala Sharma, and Drs. Julian and Myra Stern) has also furthered my knowledge of immigration-related experiences. The clinical and social insights of Dr. Purnima Mehta, my co-chair in the American Psychoanalytic Association's discussion group, "Psychoanalysis and Immigration" (December 1995–May 1998), have also helped in my thinking about matters pertaining to immigration. The presenters at the meetings of this discussion group, Drs. Regine Benalcazar-Schmid, William Kenner, Mali Mann, Peter Scou, and Hugo Zee, also enriched my knowledge of the psychosocial intricacies of immigration.

I have been deeply gratified by my collaboration with Dr. Adeline van Waning of the Dutch Psychoanalytic Society and Drs. Jelly van Essen, Mia Groenenberg, and Ildis Santini of PHAROS (Dutch Mental Health Organization for Refugees), Amsterdam, in pursuit of refining our understanding of the trauma of immigration and exile. Together, we presented some of our work at the IPA–UNESCO meetings in Lima, Peru, held in April 1998. I am thankful to Dr. Moises Lemlij of Lima, Peru, for his kind invitation. I was also extremely honored by Ambassador Nathaniel Howell's (former U.S. Ambassador to Kuwait) acting as a discussant for another panel on traumatic migrations that I chaired at the same meeting. The deep personal friendship of Dr. J. Anderson Thompson, Jr., has always been a source of pleasure, knowledge, and strength for me and I wish to acknowledge this debt here.

Dr. Michael Vergare, Daniel Lieberman Professor and Chairman of the Department of Psychiatry and Human Behavior at Jefferson Medical College, Philadelphia, provided unwavering support to my academic activities and I wish to thank him for this. I must also acknowledge the multifaceted help provided by Drs. Gregg Gorton and Steve Schwartz in my clinical and administrative activities at Jefferson Medical College. I also wish to thank Ms. Faye Landau Kahn, who was immensely helpful to me when I arrived at Jefferson Medical College twenty years ago and who has since remained a supportive friend.

Colleagues at the Philadelphia Psychoanalytic Institute have been of great importance to me and there are a few that I especially wish to acknowledge: Dr. Jennifer Bonovitz who, along with Dr. Rao Gogineni, spearheaded the Philadelphia Psychoanalytic Society's effort to bring psychoanalysis to young Southeast Asians in the Philadelphia metropolitan area; Dr. Ira Brenner, whose personal friendship over the last twenty-three years has been immensely meaningful to me; Dr. Karl Doghramji, who permitted me to quote from a personal letter he had written me years ago; Dr. Philip Escoll and Ms. Miriam Field, who allowed me to use some of their clinical material; and Dr. Steve Samuel, who gave me permission to cite some co-authored material in this book's chapter on identity.

I am extremely thankful to the patients who have given me permission to use material from my psychotherapeutic or analytic work with them. Not all clinical material, however, comes from my own practice. Drs. George Awad (Toronto), Leonard Horowitz (Topeka, Kansas), Mali Mann (Palo Alto, California), Reuben Portnoy (Philadelphia), Seymour Rabinowitz (Charlottesville, Virginia), and Elsa Ronningstam (Cambridge, Massachusetts) have graciously given me permission to use some of their clinical material as well as their personal correspondence with me. Assistance in the form of locating important references was also offered by Drs. Galina Mindlin and Alan Morrison, psychiatric residents at Jefferson Medical College, and by Ms. Panna Naik of the Van Pelt Library of the University of Pennsylvania. Drs. Peter Olsson and Pratyusha Tummala-Narra, and Ms. Sudha Singh also provided useful material for the book. To all of these individuals, my sincere thanks.

The "holding" function of my immigrant friends from the Indian subcontinent has been of deep significance in conceptualizing and presenting the ideas contained in this book. Prominent among these individuals are Nina Ahmad and Ahsan Nasratullah, Dilip Ahuja and Gayathri Arekere, Subhash and Shashi Bhatia, Atin and Lalima Bhattacharya, Subhash and Tuni Bose, Sudhir Chopra, Srilata Gangulee, Alvira Gilani, Naresh and Bubble Julka, Sukhomoy and Krishna Lahiri, Bharat and Veena Luthra, Shantanu and Rachana Maitra, Diditi Mitra, Iftikhar Nasim, Arvind and Sunanda Patel, Ramani and Suman Ramakrishnan, Mohan and Anu Rao, Azra Raza, Ram and Kalpana Shah, Shankar Vedantam, and Ashwini Tambe.

I also wish to thank two groups of individuals, one predictable and the other, on the surface, a bit curious. However, neither their predictability nor their unexpected nature diminishes the truth of my feelings. The first group is comprised of the staff at my publishing house, especially Ms. Judy Cohen, my efficient editor and sophisticated critic, and Ms. Norma Pomerantz, my source of relief for all varieties of anxieties that crop up in the course of publishing a book. I have worked with both of them on many previous books as well and my gratitude to them is deep and sustained. The second group is comprised of immigrant cab drivers in various large citities of this country. They have frequently shared their experiences of immigration with me, often in poignant details, and I wish to thank them here.

My secretary, Maryann Nevin, has been helpful to me in ways that are both explicit and subtle. She deciphered my handwriting, prepared numerous drafts of the manuscript, conducted literature searches, and, at times provided me with both the right words and the right attitude for expressing a certain idea. In simple words, she made my work easier.

Part I

IMMIGRATION

1

PSYCHOSOCIAL
VARIABLES
ASSOCIATED
WITH
IMMIGRATION

Immigration from one country to another is a complex psychosocial process with significant and lasting effects on an individual's identity. Leaving one's country involves profound losses. Often one has to give up familiar food, native music, unquestioned social customs, and even one's language. The new country offers strange-tasting food, new songs, different political concerns, unfamiliar language, pale festivals, unknown heroes, psychically unearned history, and a visually unfamiliar landscape. However, alongside these losses is a renewed opportunity for psychic growth and alteration. New channels of self-expression become available. There are new identification models, different superego dictates, and fresh ideals. One thing is clear: immigration results in a sudden change from an "average expectable environment" (Hartmann 1959) to a strange and unpredictable one.[1]

---

1. The emphasis on immigration from one country to another should not make one overlook the fact that similar issues can be faced by individuals moving to culturally diverse regions within the same country. A poignant example of such "interior migrations" (Grinberg and Grinberg 1989, p. 17) is the character played by Jon Voight in the popular 1969 movie *Midnight Cowboy*. The sociological observations of Coles (1967) on South-to-North migration in the United States and of Brody (1973) on interior migrations within Brazil are also pertinent in this regard. The New Zealand poet James Baxter (1958) has rendered his experience of moving from one to another region of his country in a beautiful poem entitled "The Return."

The mixture of pain over the losses inherent in the process and anxiety consequent upon altered external (and internal) reality mobilizes a mourning process, the outcome of which depends upon a large number of variables. I devote the major part of this chapter to a step-by-step discussion of these variables. After this I tackle certain other aspects of the immigration experience (e.g., gender, marriage, homosexuality) that have remained unaddressed in the pertinent literature. I conclude with a summary of the ideas and hypotheses presented here.

FACTORS AFFECTING THE OUTCOME

> Clearly, the immigrant must give up part of his individuality, at least temporarily, in order to become integrated in the new environment. The greater the difference between the new community and the one to which he once belonged, the more he will have to give up. [Grinberg and Grinberg 1989, p. 90]

> Since moving from one location to another involves loss—loss of country, loss of friends, and loss of previous identity—all dislocation experiences may be examined in terms of the immigrant's or the refugee's ability to mourn and/or resist the mourning process. The extent to which the individual is able intrapsychically to accept his or her loss will determine the degree to which an adjustment is made to the new life. [Volkan 1993, p. 65]

Circumstances of and Reasons for Migration

The circumstances surrounding migration and the motivations for undertaking such a major step play a paramount role in determining what psychological events will follow. Many things are involved here. *First,* whether the immigration is going to be temporary or permanent makes a big difference. The situation of a diplomat assigned for a predetermined length of time to a foreign country differs from that of the migrant who has left home in the hope of settling down in a new land. *Second,* the degree of choice in leaving one's country affects the subsequent adaptation. Also pertinent here is the time available for preparing oneself to leave a place. A sudden departure precludes anticipatory mourning and complicates subsequent adaptation. *Third,* the possibility of revisiting the home country has its own effect on the outcome of the migratory process. Those who can easily and frequently visit their countries of origin suffer less than those who are barred from such "emotional refueling" (see more about this below). *Fourth,* the reasons for leaving one's country also play a role in determining success or failure in adapting to the new environment. As regards external reality, was one "escaping from" financial hardship, political persecution, or ethnic strife, or was one "heading toward" new opportunities, wider horizons? Psychologically, was immigration an anxious or angry repudiation of primary objects or a manifestation of the ego's healthy alloplastic capacity? Often enough, if intrapsychic separation from parents is difficult

> leaving to go far away to another country can provide an illusory sense of both separation and independence. Emigration may be a way of abandoning one or both parents or even a sibling. It may serve to take revenge on a demanding or controlling parent, as well as expressing a desire to free oneself from an oppressive relationship. [Marlin 1997, p. 244]

To be sure, any sharply dichotomous view of motivations underlying migration is artificial, but the outcome of immigration might indeed vary with the economic balance of reality vs. intrapsychic and adaptive vs. neurotic components.

All this brings up the issue of the distinction between the "immigrant" and the "exile."[2] Indeed, they differ in five important

---

2. The expression "exile" has a linguistic twin in the term "refugee." The former emphasizes the inability or unwillingness to revisit the home country while the latter emphasizes the element of escape from danger or persecution (see *Webster's New Collegiate Dictionary* [1987], p. 435 and p. 991 respectively). Actually the two conditions (i.e., blocked revisiting and escape from danger) usu-

ways. *First,* the immigrant has left his country voluntarily while the exile has been forced out of his land. *Second,* the immigrant has usually had more time available for preparing to leave, while the exile has had little or no notice before his departure. *Third,* less traumatic events are generally associated with the immigrant's leaving his home; the exile has often fled a catastrophic sociopolitical situation in his country.[3] *Fourth,* the immigrant retains the possibility of revisiting his home country while the exile, having broken the "tether of belonging" (Akhtar 1992a), lacks this important source of emotional refueling. *Finally,* the manner in which the two groups are received by the host population also tends to vary. The immigrant arrives with less sociopolitical baggage and encounters greater hospitality than the exile, who is viewed with suspicion and accepted reluctantly by the host population. These external distinctions contribute to the differences in the intrapsychic processes of mourning and adaptation in the two groups (see Chapter 3).

The definition of exiles as those forced out of their country should not make one overlook the fact that the status of an immigrant can at times suddenly change into that of an exile. Because of sudden political changes in the country of their origin, immigrants may find themselves abruptly cut off from their homes. Ambassador Nathaniel Howell, who was the U.S. Ambassador to Kuwait at the time it was invaded by Iraq and who has maintained ongoing contacts with displaced and traumatized Kuwaitis, states that

> Involuntary loss of "home" is undoubtedly among the most traumatic losses that may befall an individual or a group. The loss of the associated sense of security, familiarity, and historical continu-

---

ally occur together. The term "exile" is being used here to denote both these types of severely traumatized migrants.

3. The post-Holocaust diaspora of Jews is a stunning example of traumatic migration as a result of religious persecution. Another example is constituted by the events surrounding the partition of India in 1947. In the three years that followed, ten million Hindus and seven million Muslims moved from one region to the other in response to India's bloody and tragic division along religious lines.

ity is acute even where no physical threat or actual injury is involved. Among those most severely affected by the Iraqi occupation of Kuwait, for instance, in a study carried out three years after the experience (1992–93), we found many individuals who happened to be out of their country when the aggression occurred. In-depth interviews with a representative sample of such persons revealed the trauma they experienced when they awakened in Cairo, London, or the United States to discover that they "no longer had a country." They were physically "safe" (although most had family members under brutal occupation) but their passports and currency were worthless; they found themselves literally without identity. [Howell 1999, p. 164]

This demonstrates how an individual's status can change from an immigrant to an exile. The opposite can also happen, as is evident in the situation of Eastern European Jews who left their countries in the wake of the Nazi Holocaust and became exiles and refugees in this country. With the fall of the Soviet Union and the opening up of various Eastern European countries, their psychological status has suddenly changed to that of immigrants. In other words, they now have the possibility of revisiting, indeed, relocating should they wish, to their original countries.

Matters become even more complex when the intrapsychic state of being a refugee and an immigrant coexist with each status representing a different era of one's life. For instance, an individual might migrate from one country to another as an exile or a refugee and then years later remigrate to a third country as a voluntary immigrant. The psychological vicissitudes of mourning in such cases are complicated. Often, the country voluntarily left serves as an object that can both be idealized and, more or less, mourned, while the country from which one was ejected remains devalued and pretty much unmourned in the mind.

Access to Refueling

The term *emotional refueling* was originated by Furer (quoted in Mahler et al. 1975, p. 69) to designate a toddler's frequent return to his mother from his forays in an ever-expanding outer world. The renewed perceptual input from mother recharges the internal battery of symbiotic dual unity and enhances the child's confidence. With more firm and stable internalization of the mother, the need for such contact diminishes. Also, with burgeoning ego capacities and with advance in age, the forms such refueling takes become more varied and shift from mother proper to other sources of psychic strength.

While characteristic of early childhood development, this phenomenon is of profound significance in the life of an immigrant. Separated from "motherland," the immigrant needs external reinforcement of his intrapsychic connection to her. Ideally, two sources of such support are available to him. One is actual or *extramural refueling*, which includes making international phone calls to relatives left behind and undertaking trips back to the home country. The other is *intramural refueling*, or the anaclitic support offered him by family members who have emigrated along with him and by the larger network of a homoethnic community (e.g., friends, merchants, or physicians who are co-nationals). Elsa Ronningstam (personal communication, 1997) notes that the homoethnic community may not only be a source of emotional refueling but at times can introduce immigrants to unfamiliar aspects of their own personality and culture. She states that "I was personally surprised to face new aspects of my Swedish identity, as well as totally unexpected corrective experiences in this new Swedish community here in Massachusetts."

Visiting ethnic marketplaces, celebrating one's original festivals, watching ethnic television shows, and attending services at religious centers that are operated by those from one's country of origin are among the activities that offer the immigrant an ethnopsychic rejuvenation. The renowned Greek poet, Constantine Cafavy (1906) has eloquently described this phenomenon among early Greek immigrants:

> The only thing surviving from their ancestors
> was a Greek Festival, with beautiful rites,
> with lyres and flutes, contests and garlands.
> And it was their habit toward the festival's end
> to tell each other about their ancient customs

and once again to speak Greek names
that hardly any of them still recognized.
["Returning from Greece," p. 369]

Those individuals to whom these sources are available—and
especially if they retain the possibility of revisiting the home country—fare much better in adjusting to their new circumstances.
Herein lies a major difference between the immigrant and the
exile. Unable to revisit his land of origin, the exile not only lacks
emotional refueling but also cannot update and revise the internalized pictures of his early environment. The streets, schools,
playgrounds, and homes of his childhood are lost forever. Even
the graves of his ancestors become inaccessible to him (see Akhtar
and Smolar [1998] for the significance of visiting graves). Mourning, at all possible levels, is therefore impeded and the potential
for a frozen grief becomes greater (see also Volkan 1990).

Age at Migration

Because immigration is a destabilizing process, the degree to which
psychic structure has consolidated, the extent of its continuing
reliance upon "stimulus nutriment" (Rapaport 1960) from external reality, and the conscious and unconscious fantasies active at
the time of migration can make a big difference in the later psychological adjustment. Age at the time of migration thus becomes
a very important variable. Immigrants of different age groups face
different problems. The situation with children is especially complicated. They are hardly ever immigrants in the true sense of the
word. "Parents may be voluntary or involuntary emigrants, but
children are always 'exiled': they are not the ones who decide to
leave and they cannot decide to return at will" (Grinberg and
Grinberg 1989, p. 125). Infants and toddlers can be quite deeply
affected,[4] though mostly in an indirect way, that is, through the
destabilization of the parental psychic structures. Being largely

---

4. A special situation is constituted by young children who are adopted by
individuals living in foreign countries (Norma Pomerantz, personal communi-

preverbal, children at this age depend greatly upon the affective attunement of their parents to help metabolize their inchoate internal states of emotion and thought. Anything that interferes with the "container" (Bion 1967) function of the maternal reverie tends to leave undigested residues of experience in the child's mind.[5] In the case of migration, if the parents' decathexis of the country of origin in the months before leaving and their anxiety and mourning upon arrival in the new country are profound, then the young child might lose their much needed ego support and suffer adverse consequences (Bonovitz and Ergas 1999).

Older children facing migration tend to elaborate fantasies involving the event. The parental prerogative for decisions in this realm can easily get picked up in children's oedipal fantasies. "The mother, in the boy's unconscious fantasy, emigrates to follow the father and does not consider the harm it may cause the child; the father, in the girl's unconscious fantasy, emigrates to offer security or well-being to the mother without considering the girl's suffering" (Grinberg and Grinberg 1989, p. 125).

The period of adolescence is perhaps even more tricky for migration. At this time, the individual is faced with the task of "second individuation" (Blos 1967) or an inner disengagement from the primary love objects of infancy and childhood. Such disengagement causes drive disregulation and confusion regarding one's identity. It can only be worked through if a sustained peer group with whom trial identifications, increased ego autonomy, and sexual freedom can be practiced is available. The mourning over

_____

cation 1999). Here, the loss of a familiar perceptual environment is combined with the loss of the biological parents, a dual trauma that is especially intense if the child is somewhat older and if maternal and environmental bonding has taken place.

5. Freud's childhood migrations (at age 3 from Freiberg to Leipzig, and at age 4 from Leipzig to Vienna) were not devoid of psychic impact. He "never forgot the forests around Freiberg" and his "vocal, often reiterated detestation of Vienna" (Gay 1988, pp. 9, 10) reflected not only the hardship, solitude, and anti-Semitism he faced there but perhaps also the fact that Vienna was not Freiberg!

the loss of childhood is compensated for by the peer-facilitated move toward age-appropriate identity and object relations. If the cultural platform on which such a drama is unfolding suddenly changes, the capacity for psychic development suffers. Loss of familiar cultural institutions at the very time one is fiercely exerting autonomy from parents burdens the adolescent ego with "double mourning" (van Essen 1999). The degree to which parents remain bonded with each other and stable within their individual selves can play a mitigating role in such circumstances.

All in all, it seems that, regardless of specific age

> Children's immigration experiences are to some extent attributable to their parents' attitudes. The clouds of mourning for loved ones left behind, guilt or remorse, fear of retribution for the audacious step towards independence, and anxiety about the unknown may trouble parents and blur the vision of their children. The need of parents to insulate themselves and maintain their native culture or, alternatively, their desire to become part of the dominant society, significantly affects the children. Sometimes the children bear the brunt of their parents' fear of losing their bearing. [Kahn 1997a, p. 278]

Some migrations might be manifestations of the so-called midlife crises. At the other end of the life span, during old age, there are other problems.

> An old person in general does not wish to move: it is painful to leave things that give him security; his past is much greater than his future; he always loses more than he gains. If he moves or emigrates because of adverse circumstances or to follow his children so as not to remain alone, he is very unhappy: he feels regressively dependent, like a child, but without a child's expectations and growth potential to reach new achievements. [Grinberg and Grinberg 1989, p. 128]

Ahmad (1997) points out that immigrant elders can be adversely affected by the acculturation of their younger generation. Often they come from cultures in which children were expected not only to care for their aged parents but to actually live with them. When the latter does not turn out to be true, they are sorely disappointed. Carlin (1990) presents a formidable list of problems faced by elderly refugees and immigrants. Among these are (1) isolation from former friends, (2) problems in making new friends, (3) limits on independence, (4) motility, (5) fear of failure to learn the new language, (6) not having anything useful to do, (7) disapproval by children and grandchildren, (8) feeling unneeded and unappreciated, (9) medical illnesses, and (10) facing death.[6] The last is always difficult, but it becomes even more so when one is far from the land, graves, and spirits, as it were, of one's ancestors. Facing death and burial in a land that feels foreign gives rise to deep sadness and existential shame. Bahadur Shah Zafar (1775–1862), the last Mughal King of India, who was exiled by the British, gave voice to this while awaiting death in Rangoon, Burma (now Myanmar).

> Kitna hai bud-naseeb Zafar; dafn ke liye
> Do gaz zameen bhi na mili koo-ye-yaar mein.
>
> "Cursed by the fate seems Zafar; for his burial
> he could not find two yards of land in his own country." (1862, p. 89)

All this would suggest that old age is not a suitable time to migrate, and I tend to agree. Doghramji (1994), however, offers a different perspective:

> It would seem that the best times for one to emigrate are when he is either young or old, not in between. During infancy and childhood, parents and siblings play a much greater role in development than society at large and, as long as the family emigrates as a unit, the child's support structure remains intact. Later, when latency and

---

6. At age 82 and approaching the end of his life, Freud moved from Vienna to London. Although he had detested Vienna and had left the city feeling his life threatened, the move was not entirely without pain. In Freud's own words, "the feeling of triumph at liberation is mingled too strongly with mourning, for one had still very much loved the prison from which one has been released" (Freud, letter to Max Eitingon, June 6, 1938, quoted in Gay [1988], p. 9).

adolescence are reached, one can begin the process of the assimilation of cultural identity. It is somewhat like starting to build a house and, after excavating the site, changing one's mind about the blueprint plans. This does not pose a great problem, because there is still much room for change. A larger pit can always be dug. When one is older presumably a stable sense of one's cultural, religious, and social identity has already been formed and the task at hand is that of transition within the context of a stable cultural ego. The house has already been built and cannot ever be changed too drastically. Instead, one updates the kitchen and bathrooms and adds a new family room with a cathedral ceiling. However, for the individual in his latency or adolescence years, a stable balance between id drives and the superego has not yet been fully achieved, and that process still requires a peer group and social and cultural input. Additionally, a stable cultural ego has yet to be formed since the process of its construction has just begun. Therefore, after emigration, the task at hand is akin to building a new house on an old foundation. If the old foundation does not match the new house plans, which it cannot if the new culture is too different, then the foundation itself must be revised to some extent to accommodate the new plans. The task is more difficult, which must lead to greater confusion, and a poorer adjustment for some [Doghramji, personal communication April 28, 1994]

Pre-immigration Character

It is indeed tempting to look for specific personality constellations that predispose individuals to migrate. Perhaps those who lack rootedness (schizoid individuals), possess great ambition (narcissistic individuals), love novelty in life (antisocial individuals), and those who wish to get away from persecuting others (paranoid individuals) are more prone to migrate. While this might be true, it is important to recognize that the decision to migrate emanates from a complex interplay of intrapsychic and socioeconomic factors. Characterologic traits are only one among the many variables involved.

Character organization, on the other hand, plays a much greater role in how the individual adapts to his or her new country. Menges (1959) warns that the risk of inordinate homesickness and consequent maladaptation is greater in persons who have had limited success in achieving the psychic capacity for individuation. Grinberg and Grinberg (1989), invoking Balint's (1959) concepts of "ocnophilic" (contact-seeking, object-collecting, security-minded) and "philobatic" (thrill-seeking, novelty-searching, independent-minded) types, come to a similar conclusion. In other words, they suggest that persons of the former type might experience greater difficulty in leaving their places of origin than would the latter type. My own sense is that the "ocnophil" might have more difficulty in the earlier phases of immigration but might gradually rediscover objects of attachment in the new land and séttle down. The "philo-bat," in contrast, might enjoy the freedom afforded him by his new milieu, only to become restless later on. In either case, it seems that the extent to which an individual has achieved the capacity for true, intrapsychic separateness greatly influences the degree to which he or she would be able to tolerate the moments of lone-liness that are inevitably associated with immigration.

Nature of the Country Left

The psychological outcome of immigration also depends upon the nature of the country or region one has left behind. The move from a poor to a rich country, with the inevitable financial gains, tends to mobilize unconscious guilt. Two lines of an Urdu poem I wrote in 1980, that is, seven years after my immigration to the United States, portray this very sentiment.

> Aasoodgi pe apni pashemaan se hain hum,
> Hain itne khush, ki thorey pareshaan se hain hum
>
> [Affluence asks for its own price: a puzzling remorse.
> Is happiness beginning to worry me? Of course.]

On the conscious level, such guilt is about having surpassed friends, family members, and fellow countrymen in one's material acquisitions. At a deeper level, however, lurk more personal issues of oedipal incestuous guilt and preoedipal "separation guilt" (Modell 1965).

Those who have left politically or territorially unstable regions of the world also have greater difficulty with the mourning–liberation process of immigration. An unpublished discussion of my first paper on immigration (Akhtar 1995) by Toronto-based analyst George Awad (1995) addresses this point. While acknowledging the existence of guilt in immigrants from stable nations—after all, they *chose* to leave others behind—Awad notes that

> there is another type of guilt, the "survivor's guilt" which might be more common in refugees. We feel guilty for surviving while others have not. In addition, we mourn the loss of loved ones, of the homeland, of continuity. Thus guilt and mourning are linked together and may be used defensively against each other. In fact, survivor's guilt has been far more focussed upon in the literature of the Holocaust, for obvious reasons. I think immigrants who come from troubled regions of the world, where there are continuous destruction, death, and losses need to resolve their survivor's guilt as much as they need to mourn. [Awad 1995, p. 6]

For immigrants and refugees from nations that are yet to be politically born, hope for the glorious day when their nations might achieve official statehood can impede mourning and assimilation. Doghramji (1994) states:

> There are a number of people who have been displaced from their homelands for generations and live with the hope of, someday, leaving for their own country (once it is established). Examples include the Armenians, Palestinians, Kurds, and many others. It would seem that the process of transition after emigration would be more difficult in this situation. [Personal communication April 28, 1994]

In contrast, migrating from an affluent country to a less affluent country, despite its occasional humanitarian and spiritual overtones, might itself be a manifestation of unconscious guilt; see in this connection Lapierre's (1985) *City of Joy*, which describes the migration of a North American physician to the largely poor city of Calcutta in India. Guilt is also prominent in immigrants from the state of Israel. More intensely than other immigrants, they keep believing that they will sooner or later go back to Israel. Moreover, they keep a low profile and want to avoid being seen (or seeing themselves) as defectors who abandoned the "Promised Land":

> In their homeland they would be called a *yored*, a derogatory nick-name meaning "one who descends by leaving Israel," thereby shattering the basic tenets of Zionism. This is in contrast to *oleh*, one who ascends by immigration to Israel. The *yored* is perceived as a selfish and weak person, a failure and a traitor. [Knafo and Yaari 1997, pp. 221–222]

In their illuminating essay, Knafo and Yaari highlight how "the effects of Jewish and Zionist history as well as the pressures deeply ingrained in the Israeli social structure have contributed to (these) immigrants' dilemmas" (p. 238). Besides the variety of denials described by these authors, there is the phenomenon of delayed onset of mourning regarding migration from Israel. Pnina Pinchevsky, an Israeli colleague who now lives in Montreal, describes her experience in this regard as follows:

> I am having a delayed reaction to my immigration experience. Maybe it is so delayed because during my first years in Canada there were so many exciting changes and adaptations to be made: Meeting my husband, getting married, starting a family, establishing my social work career, etc. Only while dealing with "mid-life" issues (such as my parents' declining health, my kids moving on, etc.) did I start to comprehend my losses and the price I had paid for emigrating (although, at the same time I am also aware of the trade-off and of the opportunities I had been offered by living in Canada). I also find it interesting that when I started to think of all this I decided to leave the field of social work, which here is quite practical and task oriented, and get into the field of psychotherapy, where I am constantly dealing with issues of belonging (or—more accurately)—lack of belonging. [Personal communication, June 1998]

Magnitude of Cultural Differences

The psychological outcome of immigration also depends upon the magnitude of cultural differences between the adopted and the home country. Such differences involve a wide range of dimensions, such as attire, food, language, music, wit and humor, political ideologies, degrees and varieties of permissible sexuality, extent of autonomy versus familial enmeshment, the premium upon self-assertion versus self-effacement, subjective experience of time, the extent and nature of communication between sexes and between generations,[7] and so on. Even whether a culture is more or less receptive to the immigrant's musical or poetic inclinations can make a big difference. In some cultures, humming to oneself and even singing in public is common while in others it is not. Migration from the former type of culture to the latter type can stifle the immigrant's emotional voice. In the words of the Nobel Prize winning Russian poet Joseph Brodsky (1973),

> In the republic of ends
> and means that counts each deed
> poetry represents
> the minority of the dead. [p. 136]

While all of the factors mentioned above are important, food and language especially stand out in their significance to the immigrant:

> Food takes on special relevance because it symbolizes the earliest structural link with the mother or the mother's breast. Thus the immigrant may vehemently reject the new country's local dishes and nostalgically seek out the foods of his own country. . . . [R]efuge in food [is sought] to ease his anxiety, thus recreating an idealized breast that is generous and inexhaustible, with which he tries to compensate for the many losses during the move. He usually eats those meals in the presence of co-nationals, [and] they constitute a type of memory rite. [Grinberg and Grinberg 1989, p. 79]

---

7. Immigrant parents frequently complain that their children, born in the family's country of adoption, do not listen to them. A poignant confluence of cultural, generational, and intrapsychic conflicts characterizes such scenarios. Disentangling such communicational knots, though never easy, forms an important aspect of working with immigrant patients and their families (see Chapter 4).

His own native language is perhaps even more important for the immigrant. It is his deepest and most trustworthy link to the culture that nourished him. Adopting a new language threatens his identity, which is linked to the mother tongue, and with the lullabies sung to him by his mother forms the deepest linguistic core of internalized good objects. The greater the difference between his country of origin and country of adoption in this regard, the harder it is for the immigrant to mend his lacerated self (see Chapter 3). The following poem by Nishat Akhtar, my 19-year-old daughter, eloquently portrays the resulting sense of psychic dislocation and cultural unbelonging.

> You wake up every morning to the reminder of God.
> The sun has cracked in the East once again,
> But your desire is for the West.
> And shortly after people flood the market and streets,
> The dirt begins to rise into the dry atmosphere.
> You lean on the iron railing to your balcony,
> Neglecting its intricacy.
> Overlooking the palm trees.
> Smog and overpopulation disgust you.
> One day you will leave this place, in search of something better.
> You will be surrounded by
> Spotless suburbs,
> Fresh air and
> A naively cruel ignorance of the Other.
> But you will convince yourself that you are happy.
> No longer will the indigenous call to prayer be your awakening,
> Now, it will be the tormented cries of your future,
> Lost in the color of your skin.
> And as the sun sets in the West,
> You will shed a tear,
> Longing to be back in the East.
> Immigrant.

In essence, the magnitude of cultural differences (along a wide range of dimensions) has a powerful impact upon the mourning consequent upon immigration. If the differences are great, such mourning, and subsequent adaptation, may become exceedingly difficult. A move into the United States from Canada or England, for instance, is not the same thing as one from Korea or Yemen. Settlage's (1992) observation that marked actual differences in parental personalities evoked by the immigration process put a growing child's self and object constancy to test is pertinent here. It echoes Freud's (1923) earlier warning that if the ego's identification becomes "too numerous, unduly powerful, and incompatible with each other, a pathological outcome will not be far off" (p. 30). At the same time, it should be noted that superficial similarities of culture (say, in the case of British or Canadian immigrants to the United States) do not preclude the individual's feeling like an immigrant. In Stephen Shanfield's phrase (personal communication, April 1994), Canadian nationals who have migrated to the United States are "invisible immigrants";[8] they are not readily recognized as foreign-born nationals by the host population.[9] The losses of such individuals might be subtle but they are losses nonetheless. Julian Stern, a consultant psychiatrist in England who migrated to that country from South Africa, poignantly describes the situation.

> I think that the trauma of losing my motherland was somewhat disguised by the fact that I had had an Anglocentric upbringing, that many of the textbooks I had used, and literary and cultural icons with whom I had grown up, were English and, of course, English was my mother tongue. Thus, the move to England was somewhat masked in difference and intensity which, perhaps, made some of the mourning less acute, less visible even to myself, and thus more difficult to deal with, given its disguised status. Furthermore, the fact that I slipped quite quickly into an appropriate occupational role both helped soften the blow, and also helped mystify what ac-

---

8. Interestingly, the same term has been applied by Shokeid (1988) to Israeli immigrants, who minimize their immigrant status out of guilt for having left the "Promised Land."

9. Note in this connection that while greater attention is drawn by the Indo-Pakistani, Bangladeshi, and Caribbean immigrants in England, the fact is that the majority of immigrants to the country throughout recent history have been white (Littlewood and Lipsedge 1989).

tually was a huge disruption in my life. [personal communication, June 1999]

The Chinese poet Luo Fu (1956), who moved from mainland China to Taiwan, portrays an invisible immigrant's longing to return via a beautiful visual metaphor:

> After puffing air on the window pane,
> I draw a slender boat with my finger
> And, at the end of a narrow path,
> A man's back. [p. 88]

Discussions of cultural differences affecting the adjustment of immigrants tend to focus upon East-to-West immigrants. This is unfortunate since West-to-East immigrants also face external and internal difficulties of no less magnitude. A fictional account of a British citizen's efforts to settle in Japan,[10] in Morley's (1985) *Pictures of the Water Trade*, highlights such problems. Literature on West-to-East migration is, however, meager and further investigation of this realm seems needed.[11] One fascinating avenue to take might be through the study of the lives of six Western women who received not only acceptance but fame, even greatness, after their migration to India. These include Helena Petrovna Blavatsky (1831–1891), the founder of the Theosophical movement and a longtime resident of Bombay; Annie Wood Besant (1847–1933), the British founder of the Indian National Congress; Margaret Elizabeth Noble (1867–1911), also known as Sister Nivedita, the British disciple and exponent of the Bengali mystic Swami Vivekananda; Mère Alfassa (1878–1973) who, arriving from Paris and taking on the name of Ma Aurobindo, founded a most signifi-

---

10. William Adams, who was born in Elizabethan England in 1564 and died in Japan in 1620, is believed to have been the first English speaker to reside in Japan. Interestingly, he became an advisor to the founder of the Tokugawa shogunate and was briefly a highly influential figure in Japan.

11. An exceptional account of such a move is provided by Mura (1991), a third-generation Japanese American, who went on an academic fellowship to Japan and found the experience to have deep effects on his identity.

cant spiritual mission in South India; Agnes Bojaxhiu (1910–1997), better known as Mother Theresa, who came to Calcutta from Albania; and Sonia Gandhi (1946–), the Italian widow of the assassinated Prime Minister, Rajiv Gandhi, and herself a major figure on the contemporary Indian political scene.

Reception by the Host Population

In an established group the arrival of a newcomer stirs up mixed emotions ranging from paranoid anxieties to idealization. The newcomer might be seen as an interloper who would deprive the natives of economic opportunities and life resources, or, as an unconsciously revered messianic leader who would solve the problems of the existing community. The result is prejudice and xenophobia on the one hand and excessive kindness followed by disappointment and rejection on the other. A powerful description of the former attitude can be seen in Franz Kafka's (1926) novel, *The Castle*. The animosity of the villagers toward the protagonist, a surveyor supposedly come to work in the castle, is indeed striking. Even those who promise to protect him say, "You are not from the Castle, you are not from the village, you aren't anything. Or rather, unfortunately, you are something, a stranger, a man who isn't wanted and is in everybody's way, a man who's always causing trouble" (Kafka 1926, p. 62).

Three subvariables are involved in the host population's reaction to a newcomer: (1) the nature of the existing community, (2) the particular era in which such migration is taking place, and (3) preexisting historical ties between the country of adoption and the country of origin.[12] If the host group is already made up of a large number or variety of immigrants, assimilation of the newcomer becomes easier. When the host country is largely monoethnic, the immigrant has difficulty becoming "one of them." Thus, it is easier

---

12. Actually, there are two other factors, namely (1) the magnitude of cultural differences, and (2) the bodily characteristics of the immigrant. I have already discussed the first and will address the second later in this chapter.

to become an "American"[13] in the United States, a nation of immigrants, than it may be to become, say, a Norwegian. The possibility of receiving full citizenship is also an important variable here.
Germany, for instance, is heartbreakingly discouraging to its immigrant Turkish laborers. Even those who have lived there for
generations cannot get full citizenship. The United States is much
more welcoming, even to the extent of allowing dual citizenship
with some select countries. All this has profound effects on the
immigrant's internal mourning and external assimilation.

It should also be noted that a particular era in the history of a
country might be more receptive than another era to receiving
migrants. In addition, the previously existing historical ties between
the immigrant's country of origin and country of adoption can
impact upon the reaction of the host population. Both positive and
negative results might ensue depending on the real and unconsciously embroidered nature of those ties.

The importance of the reaction of the host population to the
newcomer's self-esteem and assimilation is nowhere more clear than
in the case of African American slaves brought to the United States
from the seventeenth century onward. Their situation was devastat-
ing not only because their immigration was forced and they lacked
emotional refueling, but also because they were psychophysically
manhandled by the host population. They were used as targets of
projection and, in an act of collective "soul murder" (Shengold
1989), brainwashed to believe in their inherent racial inferiority.
Effects of the intergenerational transmission of this trauma (Apprey
1993, 1999) are of course still evident. However, the civil rights
movement of the 1960s, the subsequent "Black is beautiful" and similar esteem-building social voices, the search for heritage and legacy
(memorialized in Alex Haley's 1976 *Roots*), and the emergence (as
well as belated recognition) of national and international heroes
from within the group, are all signs of a reversal of the situation.[14]

---

13. I am sympathetic to the Latin American sentiment that the United States
has "stolen" their identity by calling themselves Americans rather than by the more
correct North Americans. This is why I have put quotation marks around the word.

14. A significant cultural boost to an ethnic community can, at times, come

Remembering Abraham's (1911) paper on the "determining power of names," the transition, in this context, from "Negro" to "Black" to "African American" seems rich with psychosocial connotations.

Experiences of Efficacy in the New Country

The extent to which one's original psychosocial role can be resumed upon immigration also affects the assimilation process (Teja and Akhtar 1981). Maintaining one's professional identity, especially when other aspects of oneself are challenged, assures an "inner continuity in change" (Lichtenstein 1963). Problems arise when, owing to the more demanding requirements in the host country or to the inherent nature of his skills themselves, an immigrant cannot resume the vocation he has practiced hitherto. Immigrant Soviet physicians in Israel, for instance, often have difficulty finding status and employment comparable to what they had in their original country and this contributes to their feeling depressed (Ritsner et al. 1993). In the United States, one can also encounter East European and South Asian physicians who have failed medical licensing examinations and are practicing at lower levels in the health-care field or even working outside it. Low self-esteem and cynicism are frequent in such situations. Many years ago, Babcock and Caudill (1958) similarly reported the situation of a Western psychoanalyst who, working for many years in Japan, had given up the practice of psychoanalysis. He found that whenever he attempted to analyze the hostile dependency on parental figures in Japanese patients, they reacted with severe depression. Noting that such depression necessitated many supportive measures, the analyst gradually began restricting his work to psychotherapy. The issue in all these instances (and other similar ones outside the field of medicine) is basically this: to feel efficacious is to live, and to feel vocationally impotent is to psychically wither away.

---

from movies that favorably portray them or their history. The Greek American and Indian American communities were thus greatly benefited by the release of *Zorba the Greek* (1965) and *Gandhi* (1982), respectively.

Birth of Children

Children born in the country of adoption tie their immigrant parents to the new land. From the moment of their birth, through preschool years, school years, and adolescence, children bring the culture at large into the family home. Young immigrant mothers especially draw information and assistance from local mothers. And, in general, parenting necessitates a greater familiarity with the local culture. Food eaten by the family begins to change after the children's arrival and the new foods are increasingly the ones belonging to the new culture. The story books read to children inevitably contain a large share of those drawn from the local reservoirs. Homogenizing television shows and, later, local music begin to populate the family's transitional space. Imbued with object-related as well as narcissistic love for their children, immigrants start to muster a smile in place of a wince when the family name is mispronounced by the kids. The fact that in most countries birth assures the right of citizenship also becomes an impetus for the immigrant parents to be forward looking. Hope appears on the horizon and makes mourning easier. On the other hand, if the children's "local" origin and behavioral style are experienced as threatening, an ethnocultural tug-of-war begins at home. Empathy for other family members suffers. Dialogue between parents and children gets derailed and the cultural difference, instead of enriching the relationship, fuels a hateful strife between generations (Mehta 1997).

SOME UNADDRESSED REALMS

A house comes into the world, not when people finish building it, but when they begin to inhabit it. A house lives only off men, like a tomb. Except that the house is nourished by the life of man, while the tomb is nourished by the death of man. [Vallejo 1923, p. 27]

In the past, conquest and enslavement were common, while nowadays migration (both voluntary and

enforced) is the predominant experience. Individuals and groups must somehow deal with this process
in all its dimensions—political, economic, cultural,
social, and psychological. [Berry 1990, p. 90]

The Role of Bodily Characteristics

To a striking degree, the immigration literature has ignored the
role of bodily characteristics in the outcome of immigration. Neither Grinberg and Grinberg's (1989) nor Elovitz and Kahn's
(1997) book has entries for "body," "color," "eyes," "epicanthic
folds," "height," "skin color," or similar terms in their indices.
Freud's (1923) dictum that the "ego is first and foremost a bodily
ego" (p. 26) seems to have gone unheeded here. The fact, however, is that the human body and immigration are related to each
other in many ways.

First, if there is a prominent difference between the bodily
characteristics of the newly arriving immigrant and that of the
natives of his country of adoption, his acceptance by the host group
is slower. This has deleterious effects upon his assimilation and
reorganization of identity. In an ironic twist to Freud's (1924)
"anatomy is destiny" (p. 178) remark, skin color and the thickness
of epicanthic folds can acquire great significance in the context of
immigration. In other words, race plays a role here. While many
other factors are involved, such "anatomical distinctions," to wryly
use another of Freud's (1925) phrases (p. 241), might also account
for the varying emotional responses of the North American population to the forced immigration of black slaves, the desperate
refuge-seeking of East European Jews, the influence of ambitious
(if colonially gaslighted) Indians, Pakistanis, and Bangladeshis—
the *Midnight's Children* of Salman Rushdie (1980)—and the recent
spate of refugees from Cuba, Haiti, Laos, Cambodia, and Vietnam.
Abbasi (1998) notes that

there can hardly be a more striking example of the negative power
of Blackness than the current plight of the Black Ethiopian Jews in
Israel. . . . These are Jews who were brought back to Israel in 1991
and were extended full citizenship. However, their condition in Is-

rael is already complicated by the development of ghettos, welfare dependence, and poor education. Even as a Jew, being Black has become a problem for these people in a country that ostensibly welcomed them home. [p. 138]

Child immigrants are especially vulnerable to discrimination based on bodily characteristics, though adults suffer too.[15] Moreover, I wish to emphasize that it is quite possible that the child's feelings, upon being emotionally deprived by his parents, are displaced onto others ("They don't like me because I am dark") or are turned against the self ("I am not good enough because I am dark"), with the skin color becoming a convenient vehicle for such defensive shifts of aggression (Jenkins 1994). The literal and the metaphorical can readily get condensed in this realm and the containing function of skin (Bick 1968) vis-à-vis internally menacing affects can easily be lost sight of.

Second, the degree to which one uses one's body and the functions it is asked to perform vary from culture to culture. A relaxed, somewhat feudal, wine-loving novelist from Peru or France becomes a subtly derided "couch potato" in North America, where athletic prowess (or at least athletic interest) is a premium ego attribute. Similarly, those who depended upon household help and domestic servants in their countries of origin have to learn to do various chores by themselves. Initial motor clumsiness might cause shame to the immigrant, and yet acquisition of new skills (e.g., changing a flat tire) results in an internal departure from earlier models of behavior. The latter, in turn, mobilize further mourning and alteration of inner psychic reality.

Third, the degree to which body parts can be exposed or, conversely, have to be covered up, varies from culture to culture. Swimming trunks and bikinis appear frighteningly permissive, even obscene, to immigrants from sexually repressive cultures in exactly

---

15. The literature's silence on this issue might be due to the fact that most contributors to immigration studies are themselves European in extraction. Unlike African and Asian immigrants, they have not experienced the anatomical dilemmas, so to speak, of immigration.

the same fashion that *purdah, chadar,* and *hijab* (of the conservative Muslim women in the Middle East), and even the *sari* of Indian and *kimono* of Japanese women appear restrictive and silly to a Western immigrant to various parts of the Eastern hemisphere.[16] The temptation to regard one form of attire and one extent of corporeal exposure as normal and the other as abnormal is indeed great in such circumstances. A practicing psychotherapist or analyst must of course work through such prejudicial attitudes within himself or herself.

Finally, the human body is involved in migration in yet another way. Not only are there literal changes in predispositions to one or the other infectious disease or nutritional imbalance as a result of migration, there might also be enhanced vulnerability, at least in some individuals, to autoimmune and psychosomatic disorders[17] following immigration.

The Impact of Gender

In my clinical as well as social experience with immigrants of diverse national and cultural backgrounds, women seem to adapt much better to immigration. Not that they do not suffer the pain of loss or have no vulnerability to nostalgia, but their overall adjustment seems to be more grounded and satisfactory than that achieved by men. Idiosyncratic dynamics of particular individuals aside, women's better adjustment to migration seems to emanate from five sources:

---

16. Female attire is usually more culture-bound and hence more easily caught up in cross-cultural confusions.

17. Frustrations are inherent in the process of immigration, being even more marked in the cases of those immigrants who remain unemployed and cannot have gratifying experiences of efficacy in the country of adoption. Under such situations, the discharge of pent-up aggression can either be outward or inward. Gaddini (1972) notes that such outward discharge occurs through striated muscles, while the "discharge on the inside takes place through the smooth muscles of the vessels and mucous membranes" (p. 191). This latter type of aggression may increase the vulnerability to autoimmune diseases and psychosomatic suffering.

First, women seem to have a greater amount and depth of affective exchange with each other than do men. They strive for "optimal closeness" (Edwards et al. 1981) rather than "optimal distance" (Akhtar 1992b, Escoll 1992) in human relationships. To use a poetic metaphor, women are oceans, free to run into each other, while men stand apart as continents. Immigrant women thus give and receive more psychic sustenance from their native counterparts than do immigrant men from theirs.

Second, motherhood, especially when recent, transcends ethnic and national boundaries, bringing young mothers in a grocery store or a quiet neighborhood street instantly together. Much cultural information gets exchanged in such encounters. The maternal ego's need to provide the baby with the most up-to-date care propels the immigrant woman to put curiosity over shame and enhances her knowledge of the local culture.

Third, children, especially when they are young, bring the culture at large to their mothers. In their efforts at bridging the gap between the culture at home with that existing outside, immigrant children "teach" their mothers about the new world surrounding them. To be sure, such efforts are typical of children even in homocultural settings, but in the immigrant situation this aspect of the child's "self-seeking" drive (Freud 1908, p. 212) comes to have a greater reparative function toward the mother.

Fourth, in just the way women have a greater sense of commitment in love relations than do men (Kernberg 1995), they seem to have a greater acceptance of their new homelands. Here my ideas are based upon those of Altman (1977), who traced women's greater capacity for contentment to an earlier event in the girl's psychosexual development, namely the shifting of her love from mother to father. "This renunciation prepares her for renunciation in the future in a way the boy is unable to match" (Altman 1977, p. 48).

Finally, in a more than merely formal bow to Freud's (1923) declaration that "the ego is first and foremost a bodily ego" (p. 26), it can be said the phylogenetically given, biological "nesting instinct" (see in this connection Bowlby [1969]) in women also prepares the groundwork for a better adjustment in their country of adoption.

Marriage and Immigration

Broadly speaking, a good marriage compensates for and a bad marriage contributes to the pains of immigration. Taking that for granted, the relationship between marriage and immigration can be seen to depend upon two other factors: (1) the temporal relationship between marriage and immigration, and (2) the ethnic and national origins of the partners.

As far as the first variable is concerned, four scenarios are possible. *First*, if marriage has occurred long before migration and the decision to migrate is more or less a mutual one, then being married can ease the turmoil of loss and adaptation. The partners can utilize their erotic and intellectual life as a buffer against the frustrations of learning new life skills. Their mutuality would create a marital-object constancy against the backdrop of which a slow modification of their individual and collective identities can take place. Having mastered the "migration" into each other's actual and internalized extended families, the partners have a prototype for assimilation. They inform each other and learn about their new culture at a comparable pace, with mutuality and playfulness.

Second, if marriage has been entered into during the immediate pre-immigration period, then, barring exceptional external realities, it is likely that anxiety over loss and psychic destabilization is being avoided. It is almost as if the partners (or at least one of the partners—most likely the one who has initiated the migration) are preconsciously aware of their brittle psychic structures and incapacity to tolerate separation and loss. Marriage, under the circumstances, is based upon hasty and poor object choice. More importantly, rather than a genuine celebration of mutuality, it serves as a manic defense against mourning. The future of such marriages tends to be at risk.

Third, a marriage during the immediate (say, less than eighteen months) post-migration period also seems to be an attempt to ward off mourning. It is as if one were replacing lost objects by quickly finding a new object. The "manic defense" (Akhtar 1995, pp. 59–60, Klein 1935, Winnicott 1935) underlying this situation is even more transparent if a newly arrived immigrant weds a native in a matter of weeks or months. Such marriages readily fall apart as the onslaught of reality and the rumblings of inner grief become undeniable over the course of time.

Fourth, if the post-migration mourning process has run its course and the immigrant has undergone considerable identity transformation and then decides to get married, the outcome seems more likely to be favorable, given that libido predominates over aggression in all other aspects of internal and external reality. Such marriages, whether with a resident of the new country or within one's homoethnic community, arise out of the individuals' deeper knowledge and acceptance of themselves and hence of each other.

This brings us to the second variable I had mentioned earlier, that is, whether the marriage is within one's own ethnic group, or with a born citizen of the country of adoption, or with a fellow immigrant from a country other than that of one's origin. Each scenario has its own vicissitudes. In the *first* instance, the continued availability of ethnolinguistic refueling (e.g., common food, language, religious festivals) can be highly beneficial. At the same time, there is a lesser likelihood of successfully letting go of the fantasy of returning to the home country, which might impede the mourning process. In the *second* instance, too, mourning can be hampered and a nostalgia-ridden ethnic self might maintain a sequestered existence if the "native" and immigrant partners do not learn about and enjoy each other's food, music, history, and rituals. If they do so, however, the result can be quite salutary. Given some resilience of psychic structure and a healthy sense of humor, such marriages can actually be quite enriching (Kahn 1997b). In the *third* instance, that is, marriages between immigrants from two different cultures (e.g., Mexico and India), the availability of a third factor (the country that both of them have adopted as their new home) for externalization of the pent-up aggression within the couple is an added benefit. It can help bond the two immigrants together and, in small doses, can be a useful maneuver.

Legal Status

Since immigration involves the crossing of national boundaries, law becomes an undeniably important variable. Psychological outcome of immigration is better if one has entered a country with proper legal permission and needed documents. "Illegal aliens" often resort to clandestine and even dangerous ways to enter their new country. Not surprisingly, they continue to suffer post-traumatic effects of their sojourn for quite some time. Lacking ordinary civil rights, they experience a deep sense of unworthiness and shame. They become vulnerable to exploitation and constantly live with real and imagined threats to their safety and survival.

Between the extremes of legal and illegal entrants to a country lie those whose situation is ambiguous. Some among this group of individuals have entered the country legally (say, as a tourist) but have let their visas lapse, extending their stays beyond the legally permissible durations. Others are refugees allowed temporary shelter in a country but not employment opportunities and other civil privileges. Many individuals from both of these groups enter the subterranean labor force, remaining underpaid and overworked. Fractured self-esteem, irritability, regressive daydreaming, and bad temper are rampant in this sub-population. Swift and definitive resolution of their civil status and not protracted bureaucratic quagmires that often engulf them, is the remedy of the social component of their anguish. It is only after that obstacle is removed that the intrapsychic work of mourning can begin.

Immigrant marriages are also affected by the legal status of the two partners. The most stark instance of this is when a marriage is undertaken for the explicit agenda of obtaining a permanent resident status. The partner who sponsors the other for a visa might feel exploited and the one who gets the visa might feel inferior and inwardly ashamed. To be sure, such propensities can be mitigated by loving feelings between them. On the other hand, these feelings might become a nidus for further marital difficulties. A related situation is when an immigrant marries someone from "back home" and brings the partner to the new country. Till the time

the latter gets a permanent visa status of his or her own, the potential for exploitation, domination, and even abuse in such marriages
is great (Prathikanti 1997).

Homosexuality and Immigration

In my earlier work on immigration (Akhtar 1995, 1999a,b), not
only did I omit the role of gender, I also failed to include the variable of homosexuality. Through further reading, clinical experience, and social exchanges with the gay community, I have since
become aware that a complex and multileveled relationship exists
between homosexuality and immigration.

First and foremost, I came across the observation in Knafo and
Yaari's (1997) paper that, owing to the stringently negative views
of them in certain cultures, homosexual individuals tend to migrate
in greater proportions than would be otherwise demographically
expectable. *Second,* in a related vein, it became known to me that
individuals who would have kept their homosexuality a secret from
others or even from themselves might become overt in their sexual
preference after migration to a more accepting culture. In other
words, migration can unmask covert homosexuality. For many
Latin American women, migration represents "a metaphorical
boundary crossing in personal development that allows homoerotic
desires and identity issues to come to light" (Gonzalez and Espin
1996, p. 590). *Third,* among the homosexual population in the
West, especially the United States, there seems to be a greater pro-
portion of heterosexually married homosexual individuals from
the third-world countries. Forced by the pressures of family and
society, such individuals might also have had children. Their life
course resembles that of the older generation of homosexuals in
the West who also had to live such socially acceptable lives. *Fourth,*
a number of divorces among third-world immigrant heterosexual
couples seem to occur because one or the other partner becomes
more comfortable with his or her hitherto suppressed homosexuality upon migration. *Fifth,* the greater flexibility in the "top" and
"bottom" roles in the North American gay community can be destabilizing for homosexual immigrants from countries where such

roles are more rigidly delegated. Manalansan (1996) has described the identity conflicts of Filipino gay men migrating to the United States. He notes that in the Philippines gay men often cross-dress, act effeminately, and attempt to pass as women. Upon their arrival in the United States, they reject the more assimilated gay Filipino American men, since the latter act more masculine. *Finally*, aim-inhibited male homoeroticism can also be affected by migration. In many third-world countries, a greater amount of physical contact among male friends (hand-holding, arms on shoulders, kissing on the cheek, etc.), with or without drinking, seems permissible without being mistaken for "homosexuality." Upon arrival in the North American or Western European countries, such individuals lose this "good" and aim-inhibited homoeroticism and may become phobic about their previous comfort in this regard. That this loss is rarely talked about makes it even more poignant.

Dreams

While the impact of external reality on the form and content of dreams is clearest in post-traumatic disorder, unresolved grief (Volkan 1981), and the onset of the termination phase of analysis (Cavenar and Nash 1976, Oremland 1973), it is established that even mundane events of day-to-day life can trigger dreams and can contribute to their manifest content (Erikson 1954, Freud 1900). In light of this, it is not surprising that immigration, with its attendant psychosocial upheaval, profoundly affects dream life.

Four such effects are discernible. *First* and foremost, exiles and refugees might have disturbing dreams regarding the traumatic events surrounding their exit from the country of origin; refugee children are especially known to suffer from nightmares (Carlin 1990, Sack et al. 1986). *Second*, there might be specific types of dreams during the immediate pre-migration period. Themes of death and rebirth, going through tunnels, loss of physical possessions, and changes in physical appearance tend to predominate at this time. *Third*, during the early post-migration phase, identity conflicts tend to give manifest content to dreams. A young man who had recently moved from Israel to the United States, for instance, kept dreaming that he was living on an island in a trailer house with wheels under it (Portnoy 1999, personal communication). Other scenarios of not belonging anywhere completely (Meaders 1997) or desperately trying to return home but finding oneself hindered by obstacles (Marlin 1997) might also begin to appear in dreams. With resolution of identity conflicts, a gradual shift in the content of dreams tends to occur; the nighttime operas now begin to depict the emergence of the immigrant's bicultural self. While such dreams can be viewed as "state of affairs dreams" (Fairbairn 1952) or "self-state dreams" (Kohut 1977), the dynamics of wish fulfillment are of course concurrently active in their formation. *Finally,* while recent immigrants tend to revert to their mother tongue in the dream life, with increasing acculturation spoken words of the newly acquired language also start to make their appearance in dreams. Evidence of even deeper assimilation comes when visual puns and metaphors derived from the newly learned language begin to appear. A Pakistani lawyer residing in the United States for about fifteen years dreamt, for instance, that she was standing on a balcony with a wet towel in her hand that she then allowed to drop to the ground. Feeling puzzled about the dream, she reported it in her psychotherapy. Her associations revealed that she had been attempting to change a very difficult reality and was beginning to give up the struggle. In other words, she had "thrown in the towel." Since there was no such expression in her mother tongue, the visual depiction of a construct from her adopted language was indeed striking.

The Changed Man–Animal Relationship

Immigration can also alter people's relationship to animals. This is especially true of migration from predominantly agrarian societies to industrialized nations, but it is also valid for migrations from rural areas to large cities within the same country. In rurally based societies, the psychosocial distance between man and animals is significantly closer than it is in the industrialized nations. Animals of all varieties—cows, buffaloes, horses, donkeys, cats, dogs, camels, monkeys, snakes, spiders, butterflies, and even elephants, bears, and tigers—can form a part of people's everyday existence. They become receptacles of mythic projections, containers of unexpressed personal emotions, carriers of phallic exhibitionism, providers of maternal soothing, targets of dark eroticism, and brotherly companions in the journey of life (Akhtar and Brown 1999, Akhtar and Volkan 1999a,b, Freeman in press). When an individual thus raised moves to a country where contact with animals is limited to the possession of pets or visits to the local zoo, something subtle but of paramount importance is lost from his subjective experience. While I am referring to a more pervasive loss of contact with animals here, the fact that individual pets often get left behind at the time of migration should not be overlooked.[18] The resulting environmental discontinuity taxes the ego's capacity for temporal continuity, and the pain, unknown to the natives of the adopted country, goes unnoticed.[19] The frequent use of animal metaphors by immigrant poets from the so-called third-world countries testifies to the subterranean existence of such pain. Walking through the aisles of a grocery store, the Indian–North American poet Panna Naik asks:

"Milk is 'fortified, homogenized,
pasturized, and vitamins added.'
How do the cows feel, I wonder?" [personal communication, 1999]

---

18. Of course, this does not have to be the case. Freud's dogs traveled with him when he had to migrate from Vienna to London in his old age (Gay 1988). A more powerful testimony to retaining relationships with pets while migrating is evident in the instance of the psychoanalyst Dominic Mazza (personal communication, 1999). Born and raised in the rural community of Scranton, Pennsylvania, Mazza entered psychoanalytic training in cosmopolitan Washington, D.C. Throughout his fifteen-year stay there, he had a sense of being an immigrant. When he decided to move back to Scranton, he dug up the grave of his dog, a Doberman named Damien, and reinterred the remains in the backyard of his house in Scranton.

19. Alexander Solzhenitsyn (1969), until recently himself an exile, has put it this way: "Nowadays we don't think much of a man's love for an animal, we laugh at people who are attached to cats. But if we stop loving animals, aren't we bound to stop loving humans too?"

Portraying the anguish of poor and unemployed migrants, the Colombian–North American poet, Carlos Castro Saavedra (1986) evokes a deeply cynical image:

> Out of work
> Just like those dogs
> Who silently urinate on the corners of the world. [p. 94]

And, Indran Amirthanayagam (1995), a North American immigrant poet from Sri Lanka, wistfully laments the loss of her childhood playmates:

> What happened to the elephants?
> The conversation goes on and on
> What happened to the elephants
> and Rangoon, where does the rhino roam?" [p. 37]

The different ways in which a particular animal is viewed in the immigrant's two different cultures (for instance, the owl is regarded as stupid in India and wise in the United States) also burdens the ego. This shifts the nature of projections contained by the animal. As a result, the linguistic ploys of curses and endearments involving it also suffer the fate of confusion, contradiction, and atrophy.

It should also be acknowledged, however, that animals can play a helpful role in the process of migration. The company of pets during migration can indeed be quite soothing. Also, in circumstances when one suddenly becomes an exile within one's own country—*emigration without leaving home* (Kahn 1997c, p. 255, emphasis added)—animals can play a highly significant symbolic role in stabilizing the psyche. Volkan (1976), for instance, notes that when Cypriot Turks were confined in enclaves surrounded by their enemies between 1963 and 1968, they created a symbol, a parakeet in a cage, that represented their imprisoned selves. Thousands of such birds were taken as pets by them. It was as if as long as the birds sang happily the Cypriot Turks could maintain hope that they would one day regain their freedom.

SUMMARY

Only those who hate their own self, family, and culture, can want to abandon them. To become American, it must be I who becomes American. My Latin spirit must survive, because it is part of me. I want to maintain my culture, the importance of friendship, the expression of affection, and the sense of history, common among Latins and essential for social progress. [Sabelli 1997, p. 175]

This chapter emphasizes that immigration is a complex psychosocial process with a powerful impact upon an individual's identity. It notes that migrations can be from one country to another or from one culturally distinct region of the same country to another. Both mobilize a destabilization–restabilization process vis-à-vis the psychic structure. This chapter has elucidated the variables that govern the outcome of such a process. Ten such variables are identified. These include (1) circumstances and reasons for migration, (2) access to refueling, (3) age at migration, (4) pre-immigration character, (5) nature of the country left, (6) magnitude of cultural differences, (7) reception by the host population, (8) experiences of efficacy in the country of adoption, (9) intercultural marriages, and (10) birth of children in the new land. Some other areas that have remained largely unaddressed in the immigration literature are also discussed. These include (1) the role of bodily characteristics, (2) the impact of gender, (3) marriage and immigration, (4) legal status, (5) homosexuality and immigration, (6) dreams, and (7) the changed man–animal relationship as a result of immigration. Keeping this complex tapestry of factors underlying the identity change consequent upon immigration in mind, we are now prepared to examine the concept of identity itself.

Part II

IDENTITY

2

DEVELOPMENT, PHENOMENOLOGY, AND CLINICAL RELEVANCE OF IDENTITY

The concept of identity, coined by Tausk in 1919, has occupied an ambiguous place in psychoanalysis and psychiatry. A construct that is both intrapsychic and interpersonal, identity has been ambivalently held in psychoanalytic theory. Moreover, since its phenomenological constituents have not been explicitly spelled out, the concept has lacked widespread usage in descriptive psychiatry. Despite such handicaps, the concept has survived in both traditions, a testimony to its clinical significance, especially in regard to severe personality disorders. Not surprisingly, then, it is in the context of a combined psychoanalytic-psychiatric focus on borderline personality (Grinker et al. 1968, Gunderson and Singer 1975, Kernberg 1967), an illustration par excellence of severe character pathology, that the concept of identity has freshly reappeared in the clinical limelight. The recently increased interest in working psychodynamically with immigrants, refugees, and culturally diverse populations in general (Akhtar 1995a, Fischer 1971, Freeman 1997, Holmes 1992, Kakar 1985, Pérez Foster et al. 1996, Roland 1996, Taketomo 1989) has also given impetus to a reconsideration of identity as a psychic structure. A thorough explication of its development and phenomenology is, however, still lacking. My aim here is to fill this gap by synthesizing the scattered literature on identity. Although a wide range of intellectual disciplines (e.g., sociology, philosophy, anthropology) do offer insights regarding this concept, my focus is on the largely clinical perspectives of psychiatry, psychoanalysis, and clinical psychology.

I will begin by highlighting the historical evolution of the concept of identity. Then I will summarize the literature on the developmental origins of identity. Following this, I will present a composite portrait of the concept, taking into account its various phenomenological facets. I will then highlight its clinical relevance and conclude with a brief discussion of the ways to assess consolidation or impairment of identity.

HISTORICAL EVOLUTION OF THE CONCEPT

> In their search for a new sense of continuity and sameness, adolescents have to refight many of the battles of earlier years, even though to do so they must artificially appoint perfectly well-meaning people to play the role of adversaries; and they are ever ready to install lasting idols and ideals as guardians of a final identity. [Erikson 1950b, p. 261]

> The sense of identity, or awareness of identity involves comparison and contrast—with some emphasis on basic likeness, but with special attention called to obvious unlikeness. [Greenacre 1957, p. 132]

The early literature of descriptive psychiatry, especially that pertaining to the phenomenology of various psychoses, portrays many types of identity disturbances. These include the subjective experience of being someone other than oneself, being more than one individual, being an animal—the delusion of "zoophilic metamorphosis"—and being a supernatural creature or God (Batchelor 1969, Bleuler 1908, Diefendorf 1921, Fish 1964, Hinsie and Campbell 1975, Slater and Roth 1969, see also Akhtar and Brown 1999). Interest in multiple personality, currently termed Dissociative Identity Disorder (*DSM-IV* 1994, pp. 484–487), also implicitly invoked the concept of identity though the terms usually employed were "split personality," "splitting of awareness," "double consciousness," and so on (Breuer and Freud 1893–1895, Janet 1907, Prince 1905). Similarly, some of the early descriptive character typologies, for example, "morbid liars," "criminals by impulse," "professional criminals," and "morbid vagabonds" (Kraepelin 1905) seemed clearly based upon the core identity of the individuals involved. However, the term identity itself did not come up in these systems.

It was in 1919 that Tausk introduced the term into the psychoanalytic literature. Tausk examined how the child discovers his self and asserted that man must, throughout life, constantly find and experience himself anew. Freud used the term "identity" in a technical sense only once (Guttman et al. 1980). This was in his address to B'nai B'rith, where he spoke of his "inner identity" (Freud 1926a, p. 274) as a Jew. However, his infrequent usage of the specific term does not mean that a number of his ideas are not of great significance to the concept. This is especially so because he used the term *das ich* (translated into English as *the ego*) in two different ways: as an executive agency of the mind, and as the "person's self as a whole" (Strachey et al. 1923, p. 7). This latter conceptualization seems to overlap what is now termed *identity*. One can thus discern what might have been Freud's stance regarding identity by scrutinizing some of his central hypotheses regarding the ego.

> In the process of a child's development into a mature adult there is a more and more extensive integration of his personality . . . [1921, p. 18] . . . the ego is first and foremost a bodily ego. [1923, p. 26] . . . the character of the ego is a precipitate of abandoned object-cathexes and . . . it contains the history of those object choices. [1923, p. 29] . . . the ego ideal is . . . the heir of the Oedipus complex. [1923, p. 26] . . . Anatomy is Destiny. [1924, p. 178] . . . all human individuals, as a result of their bisexual disposition and of cross-inheritance, combine in themselves both masculine and feminine characteristics. [1925, p. 258]

To be sure, the word *identity* does not appear here, yet these brief statements, coupled with his B'nai B'rith declaration, succinctly portray Freud's implicit view of the genesis and consolidation of identity. This view is a comprehensive one and accommodates somatic underpinnings, gender differences, early identifications, the role of the Oedipus complex and its resolution, the ongoing synthetic function of the ego, and the ethnic and moral dimensions of character. What remained implicit yet palpably present in Freud was to be developed by his followers, though after a few decades of relative lack of interest in the concept of identity.

In the 1950s, Erikson (1950a,b, 1956, 1958) resurrected the term in his contributions to character formation. Erikson (1959) used the term *ego identity* to denote "both a persistent sameness within oneself (selfsameness) and a persistent sharing of some kind of essential character with others" (p. 12). He later dropped the "ego" prefix, in part to accommodate Hartmann's (1959) differentiation between ego and self. Erikson (1956) emphasized that identity could have many connotations and could refer at one time to "*a conscious sense of individual identity*; at another to an unconscious striving for *a continuity of personal character*; at a third, as a criterion for the silent doings of *ego synthesis*; and finally, as a maintenance of an inner *solidarity* with [the] group's ideals and identity" (p. 102, original italics).

While he noted that identity formation is a lifelong development, with its roots going back to the earliest self-recognition, Erikson emphasized the period of adolescence in the consolidation of identity. He saw the adolescent as attempting to integrate what he knew of himself and his world into a stable continuum of past knowledge, present experiences, and future goals in order to elaborate a cohesive sense of personal feeling. Failure in this task led to a chaotic sense of personhood, both in its subjective and social sense.

Although Erikson's terminology gained wide acceptance and his pioneering work gave considerable impetus to the psychoanalytic study of identity, there did remain areas that needed further clarification. These included the relative significance of infantile and adolescent phases in identity consolidation, the distinctions between the usual identity crisis of adolescence and identity diffusion, and finally the correlation between the latter syndrome and the more traditional classifications of character pathology. Jacobson (1954), Kernberg (1975 1976 1980), Mahler (1958a,b, 1967), and Mahler and colleagues (1975) later recognized these limitations and attempted to fill the lacunae.

DEVELOPMENTAL ORIGINS OF IDENTITY

> Passing through many frustrations, disappointments, failures, and corresponding hostile experiences of envy, rivalry and competition, the child eventually learns the difference between wishful and more or less realistic and self and object-images. Thus not only the loving but also the hostile components of the infantile self and object directed strivings furnish the fuel that enables the child to develop his feelings of identity. [Jacobson 1964, p. 61]

> Different childhood periods determine different integrations of ego identity, and the general integration of ego identity stemming from all these partial ego identities normally operates as an attempt to synthesize them into an overall harmonious structure. [Kernberg 1976, p. 32]

Any attempt to trace the developmental origins of identity is complicated by two factors. *First*, the term *identity* has had a checkered history. Psychoanalytic theory especially has held the concept ambivalently, most likely because of its hybrid nature. Far from being purely an intrapsychic construct, identity has unmistakable social referents. Thus it borders on areas where psychoanalytic theory traditionally has been at its weakest, though with the recent emergence of an intersubjective emphasis (Dunn 1995, Hoffman 1992, Ogden 1995, Stolorow and Atwood 1989) in its various conceptualizations, this might be subject to some rectification. *Second*, various authors address various phases of identity consolidation (e.g., infancy, adolescence), utilize various methodologies, (e.g., child observation, deductive theorizing, analytic reconstruction), and even use varying terms (e.g., identity, self, and, in Freud's case, even ego). As a result, the comparability of their work and the pooling together of their observations might be questionable. Moreover, disagreements do exist in this area and much uncertainty still persists regarding many of these matters. The synthesis offered here then is just that: a synthesis. Its aim is to present something of a consensus view of identity development, while also indicating areas of disagreement. It will emphasize that identity consolidation is an ever-evolving process that begins before the birth of the individual and continues throughout the life span, even during senescence.

The Seeds of Identity before Birth

The origins of a child's identity can be traced backward not only to the earliest days of his infancy but to even before his actual birth. Two factors begin laying ground for what will be the child's *basic core* (Weil 1970): the baby's genetic blueprint, and the parental wishes for and expectations of the coming baby.[20] The former provides the hard-wired psychomotor proclivities, that is, *temperament* (Thomas and Chess 1977, 1984), that enter into a dialectical play with the early environmental inputs. The latter affect the way in which the newborn will be psychologically "held" (Winnicott 1965) in maternal attention. Here the specific family myths, conflictual wishes on the part of the parents, and intergenerational transmission of traumatic events play an important role in the future child's identity formation. In this connection, it is significant to note that the parents' mourning–liberation process in immigration can have a significant impact upon their offspring's core self-representation. Children born earlier in the course of immigration might suffer more than those born when the parents are more advanced in their intrapsychic work of mourning and adaptation.[21]

---

20. For a somewhat different perspective on this matter, especially as it involves the actual intrauterine life, see Piontelli (1987, 1988).

21. Also, of course, the younger children have the advantage of learning from older siblings born and raised in the new culture.

Another such instance is constituted by a child conceived soon after the loss of a significant person in the mother's life (e.g., a loved parent). Such a child might become unconsciously equated in the parental psyche with the deceased. This occurrence is by no means ubiquitous and is seen mostly in association with unresolved grief in the mother (Volkan 1987). Under such circumstances, the psyche of a "replacement child" (Cain and Cain 1964, Poznanski 1972) is the recipient not only of the mother's expectable wishes but also of the "deposited representations" (Volkan 1987) of the mother's earlier love object. He is therefore vulnerable to a dichotomous identity with potentially contradictory demands on the ego throughout his life. With the birth of the child, these potentialities acquire a realistic shape, often encoded in the first name the child is given (Abraham 1911).

Early Childhood

The human infant arrives in the world preadapted for participating in human interactions (Emde 1983, Stern 1985). Among the capacities that are present at birth and that facilitate such interactions are "a propensity for participating in eye-to-eye contact; a state responsivity for being activated and soothed by human holding, touching, and rocking; and a propensity for showing prolonged alert attentiveness to the stimulus features contained in the human voice and face" (Emde 1983, p. 171).

Such "social fittedness" (Emde 1983, p. 171) of the infant has a counterpart in the mother as well. She directs speech and gestures to her infant in a simple and repetitive pattern. But more important in the development of identity is that the mother conveys a particular theme to her newborn. "The mother imprints upon the infant not an identity, but an identity theme. This theme is irreversible, but it is capable of variations, variations that spell the difference between human creativity and a '*destiny neurosis*'" (Lichtenstein 1961, p. 208, original italics). Juxtaposed to the driving pressure of this identity theme is a longing to abandon the human quality of identity altogether. For this, Lichtenstein (1961, 1963) proposes the term "metamorphosis." He sees identity and metamorphosis as incompatible but complementary since human life exists in oscillation between these two extremes.[22]

A different though not entirely dissimilar oscillation in early identity is described by Mahler (1958a,b, 1967, Mahler et al. 1975). As she observed the human infant crawl out of the psychobiologic shell of normal autism into the psychic envelope of symbiotic relatedness with the mother, Mahler also laid the groundwork for observing a potential tension between identity loss by regression into autism and identity maintenance (albeit in an enmeshed form) via human symbiosis. More significantly, Mahler traced the steps that the infant must take out of such symbiosis in order to develop his psychic separateness and individuality. These steps—differentiation, practicing, rapprochement, and "on the road to object constancy"—collectively constitute the process of separation-individuation. This process begins around 5 to 6 months of age and lasts until about 30 to 36 months of age, though its last subphase is somewhat open-ended. Passing through the differentiation (from 5 to 9 months) and practicing (from about 9 to 18 months) subphases, the child demarcates his own psychic self from that of his mother. Such separateness becomes evident through the child's emerging capacity for self-recognition both in the mirror and in

---

22. Bach (1985) later correlated such oscillations between subjective and objective self-awareness with the vicissitudes of the separation-individuation process. He pointed out that individuals who have difficulty experiencing themselves subjectively *and* objectively at the same time also experience the chronic dilemma in terms of "self-love or object-love, of isolation or merger, of sadism or masochism, and [that this] is accompanied by a mirroring (controlling) transference or by an idealizing (submissive) transference. The sadomasochism, of course, reflects the fact that the object line of rapprochement overlaps with the instinctual line of anality, and the coercion of the object serves to reduce or deny the awareness of separation" (p. 71). Besides etiologically correlating the oscillations between internal and external self-experience with the works of Balint (1968), Kohut (1977), and, most importantly, Mahler and colleagues (1975), Bach describes in eloquent detail the painful handicaps in the love and work life of "the patient [who] can either be lost in an absorbed state without being aware of himself or [who] is constantly aware of himself without being able to lose himself" (p. 72).

the use of personal pronouns that begins around this very time—that is, 18 to 21 months of age (Emde 1983, Lewis and Brooks-Gunn 1979). The strengthened sense of himself is also manifest in the child's becoming able to describe his own behavior at around 20 months of age (Kagan 1981). The separateness, however, also inaugurates the rapprochement subphase (from about 18 to 24 months) during which the child ambivalently asserts his newfound selfhood and anxiously clings to the mother for reassurance. With the continued emotional availability of the mother, these vacillations gradually settle down. This helps bring together the child's contradictory self images (e.g., passive, dependent "lap baby" and the exuberant, joyous, and self-assured toddler; or hostile and loving self-representations, etc.) into a composite whole. The attainment of self-constancy establishes a coherent, single self-representation with minimal fluctuations under drive pressures; this is the birth of identity. The parallel attainment of object constancy is characterized by the consolidation of a deeper, more sustained internalized representation of the mother, positive attachment to which is not seriously compromised by temporary frustrations.

Mahler's observation that a consolidated sense of self first emerges around 18 to 20 months of age is challenged by Stern (1985). He posits that infants begin to experience a "sense of an emergent self" (p. 37) from birth, are inherently aware of self-organizing processes, and do not enter the world in a state of self–other undifferentiation. He places the beginnings of the "sense of core self" between 2 to 6 months, that is, much earlier in time than Mahler. Stern also questions whether the self arises out of a mother–infant symbiotic matrix or whether the sense of (and even the capacity for) merger-like experiences is itself dependent upon having a separate sense of self. Lewis and Brooks-Gunn (1979), Emde (1983), and Kagan (1981), on the other hand, side with Mahler in placing the emergence of a reasonably coherent self at around 18 to 20 months of age. Mahler's views are also complemented by those of Jacobson (1954) and Kernberg (1975, 1976, 1980), which focus upon the processes of early internalizations and their intrapsychic, structure-building vicissitudes.

Jacobson introduced the terms "self-representation" and "object-representation" (endopsychic images of the self and its objects, respectively), which highlighted the fact that the phenomena involved in identity formation were ultimately intrapsychic and not interpersonal. Jacobson further proposed a fused self–object representation as the first intrapsychic structure, out of which emerges the capacity for the distinguishing self- and object-representations as separate. Still later, the mending of contradictory (libidinal and aggressive) self-representations gives birth to a coherent identity. Jacobson's views were further developed by Kernberg, who formulated a three-step process of identity formation, with a sequential increase in the later steps as development proceeds. In other words, the first of these steps is more often associated with early childhood, the second with later childhood, and the third with adolescence. It is only for didactic ease that the three steps are presented together in this section on early childhood.

The *first* step in Kernberg's process is introjection, whereby certain affectively charged, specific attributes of others are internalized without being fully assimilated into the self-image. Such "an organized cluster of memory traces" (Kernberg 1976, p. 29) includes an object image, a self-image, and the affective coloring of the interaction binding the self and the object. The *second* step is identification, which implies a less concrete and more role-oriented internalization of significant others in relationship to oneself. Identifications, unlike introjects, do not feel like a "foreign body" in the self; topographically speaking, identifications are situated "deeper" in the self-system than introjects, which in their experiential aspects are often preconscious. Clearly, a more sophisticated ego, with more advanced cognitive and perpetual abilities, is involved in identification than in introjection. The *third* step is identity formation, whereby diverse identifications are synthesized into a harmonious gestalt. In this process, individual identifications become "depersonified" (Jacobson 1954)—that is, they lose their concrete similarities with their original sources. This selective repudiation and mutual assimilation of earlier identifications leads to a new psychic configuration, the ego identity.

Later Childhood

The "constitutionally predestined gender-defined differences in the behavior of boys and girls" (Mahler et al. 1975, p. 224) get psychologically elaborated as the child gains an awareness of the distinction between the two sexes (Freud 1925). This traditionally held developmental view is challenged by the observations of Galenson and Roiphe (1971), who propose that genital sensations of a vague, internal type and of a localized, external type (in girls and boys respectively) begin even earlier and contribute to the subtle differences in the separation-individuation process of the two sexes (Olesker 1990). It is, however, during the phallic-oedipal phase of development that body-image representations emerge from pregenital libidinal positions and bisexual identifications to firm up the foundations of future sexual identity.

The Oedipus complex now appears on the scene. Libidinal strivings of both a "positive" (toward the opposite-sex parent) and "negative" (toward the same-sex parent) type develop. The renunciation of positive oedipal desires establishes an incest barrier in the psyche and lays the structural foundation (superego) for all subsequent morality. The child's acceptance of the chronological lag between his or her oedipal longing and the attainment of adult genital capacity deepens the acceptance of reality in general. The resulting narcissistic injury is compensated for by the projection of infantile narcissism onto the parents (especially the same-sex parent) and the formation of the ego ideal. This structure implies both hope and future, and it therefore facilitates the child's "entrance into a temporal order" (Chasseguet-Smirgel 1985, p. 28). These developments are accompanied by the child's acquisition of generational filiation (being a son or daughter, not merely a boy or girl) and, through that, a sense of historical continuity. Identity now gains the facet of belonging to a group, that is, the family of origin, and, by extension, to similar families. The resulting identifications along the lines of "us" and "them" yield cultural and ethnic dimensions to the self-experience.

With the passage of the Oedipus complex, the relatively quiet phase of "latency" is ushered in. The exercise of burgeoning motor and cognitive skills furthers secondary narcissism and strengthens the sense of who one is and what one can do. Identity remains more or less certain during this period.

Adolescence

It is during adolescence that the issue of identity is once again brought to the surface with full force. While psychological separateness had so far depended upon a secure internalization of the parental homeostatic functions (Freud 1923, Mahler 1958a,b, 1967, Mahler et al. 1975, Settlage 1991), acquisition of such separateness in adolescence requires a reverse process; this is the *second individuation process of adolescence* (Blos 1967). Emotional disengagement from the internalized early object becomes necessary at this stage, and this, coupled with the characteristic drive upsurge of this period, results in a certain ego instability. Progressive and regressive trends alternate, at times with disturbing rapidity. Regressive trends cause clinging to earlier modes of self-expression. Progressive trends, both defensive and autonomous, herald new self-configurations. On the one hand there is insistent disengagement from the earlier parental dictates internalized in the form of superego. On the other, there is an equally tenacious reliance upon the values of the peer group. Trial identifications and role experimentations within the latter context, coupled with the "holding environment" (Winnicott 1965) of a resilient family, gradually broaden ego autonomy and impart a greater sense of inner solidity, constancy, and abstract morality.

Gender-related differences in identity development again become evident during adolescence (Blos 1967, Fischer and Fischer 1991, Money and Ehrhardt 1972). Since adolescence fosters regression, both boys and girls retreat from oedipal conflicts and struggle with issues of control, autonomy, gender identity, and optimal distance from significant others. For the boy, the door to regressive closeness with mother is barred because it threatens his gender identity. He turns to his father and even more forcefully to his male peers for patterning his social identity. For the girl, regression to a close tie with the mother, with its attendant push–pull tensions, is more frequent. Both boys and girls alike deal with the resurgence of oedipal conflicts, but regression in object-relatedness is more frequently seen in girls.

Adolescence is also the time when sexual identity is consolidated. Renunciation of sexual aims toward primary love objects, reconciliation of active and passive sexual aims, and further synthesis of bisexual identifications facilitate this development (Blos 1967). Blos, whose work (1967, 1984) is enormously important in shedding light on these processes, suggests that it is only during adolescence that the negative oedipal strivings are truly given up. Such renunciation of homoerotic desires not only sharpens heterosexuality but also contributes prominently to the psychic image of the kind of person one aspires to become. Indeed, Blos (1984) declares that "the adult ego ideal is the heir of the negative Oedipus complex" (p. 319).

Before proceeding to the next phase of identity development (namely, adulthood) it is warranted to briefly discuss the father's role in the genesis and consolidation of identity. This is especially because the discussion so far has remained focused on the mother–child interaction.

The Father's Role

Freud (1930) declared that he "can not think of any need in childhood as strong as the need for a father's protection" (p. 72). However, for the following two decades, psychoanalytic developmental theory did not pay adequate attention to the father's role in child development. Then, in 1951 Loewald emphasized the degree to which, for a child of either sex, the father's role was a powerful force against the threat of reengulfment by the mother. Mahler and Gosliner (1955) pointed out the father's role in development of the ego and of superego precursors in the child. Greenacre (1966) observed that the overidealization of the male analyst and of analysis frequently reflected the important role of the father in the first two years of the child's life. Mahler (1967) agreed with this and emphasized that the child reacted to the father as a "breath of fresh air," one who was different from the mother and more playful. Benedek (1970) addressed the ego-building influence of the "father's identification with his child and . . . the father's identification with his own father" (p. 173). Benedek states that "it is pertinent to recall the influence that the father's changing position within his family exerts upon the personality development of his children, especially upon his sons" (p. 176). Abelin (1971), who worked with Mahler, introduced the concept of early *triangulation* as he described the role of the father during the preoedipal years of the child's development. Abelin reported child observations that revealed the ego-building, noncompetitive (in the boy) and nonerotic (in the girl) role of the father.

In a series of contributions spanning two decades, Blos (1962, 1965, 1967, 1974, 1985) demonstrated that the early, preoedipal son–father relationship critically affects the boy's self and world view for a lifetime. The little boy seeks father's approval and praise, and if these are found, a deep and lasting bond is established between them. Father's approval instills in the son "a modicum of self-possession and self-assertion—distilled, as it were, out of mutual sameness or shared maleness—which renders the wider world not only manageable and conquerable but infinitely alluring" (Blos 1985, p. 11). At the end of adolescence, father's affirmation of his son's manhood allows the latter to assume adult prerogatives. Blos noted that the last psychic structure to crystallize is the ego ideal, and that this happens as a result of renouncing negative oedipal strivings at the end of adolescence. A young man must replace his tender and submissive ties to his protective father by his own sense of ideals and moral injunctions. Ross (1979) comprehensively reviewed the literature on the father's developmental contributions, adding significant insights of his own. He posited the concept of the "Laius complex" (1982), that is, father's hostile competitiveness with his son, elucidated the dialectics of distance and intimacy in the developmental dialogue between fathers and daughters (1990), traced the vicissitudes of men's need for father figures over the life span (1994), and noted that escape from a forbidding pa-

ternal transference upon a spouse is often the unconscious mo-
tive for male infidelity in long marriages (1996).

I (Akhtar 1995b) recently summarized the multifaceted role of
father in child development as consisting of the following four
tasks:

> (1) By being a protective, loving, and collaborative partner to the
> mother, the father facilitates and enhances her ability to devote
> herself to the child. (2) By offering himself as a relatively neutral,
> ego-oriented, new object during the rapprochement subphase of
> separation-individuation, the father provides the child with stabil-
> ity, a haven from conflict, and (in the case of a boy) an important
> measure of "dis-identification" (Greenson 1968) from the mother.
> (3) By appearing on the evolving psychic horizon of the child as
> the romantic partner of the mother, the father helps consolidate
> the child's capacity to experience, bear, and benefit from the tri-
> angular familial relationship and the conflicts attendant upon it.
> (4) By presenting himself as an admirable model for identification
> to his son and by reflecting the budding femininity of his daughter
> with restrained reciprocity, the father enriches his children's gen-
> der identity and gives direction to their later sexual object choices.
> [p. 77][23]

All this results in a powerful impact on both the ego and superego, especially in the realm of disengagement from mother, language organization, modulation of aggression, establishment of
the incest barrier, acceptance of generational boundaries, capacity to respect and idealize elders, entry into the temporal order,
and, through it, a deeper sense of familial and ethnic affiliation. It
is with this backdrop that we can now take a close look at the cultural and subcultural variations in the father's contribution to his
child's growth.

With this rounded-off picture that takes into account the role
of both parents in the origins and consolidation of a growing child's

---

23. Cultural variations in the degree and manner of the father's execution
of these tasks might indeed exist. This is, however, a little-studied area and needs
further investigation.

identity, we can now resume our longitudinal survey of identity development and address its further refinements during the adult life.

Elaborations of Identity during Adulthood

While a very significant consolidation of identity does occur during adolescence, it would be erroneous to assume that identity development ceases at this point. Subsequent life tasks (for example, separation from parents and home; engagement and marriage; career choice, often requiring the overcoming of ambivalent ties to one's mentors; becoming a parent oneself) also revive conflicts regarding identity and thus provide opportunities for reworking identity-related issues. Becoming a parent is especially notable as a turning point (Colarusso 1990, 1997). The emotional challenges of raising children tax object constancy and, therefore, have an impact upon identity. On the one hand, passing one's name and psychobiological features to one's offspring consolidates the inner sense of generational lineage and continuity, thus strengthening identity. On the other, in being the recipient of a child's rapprochement subphase turbulence, the mother especially has to modulate her own reciprocal drives and contradictory object representations of the child. Here maternal object constancy comes to serve the "container" (Bion 1967) function for the child's contradictory affects, scattered self-representations, and vacillating object ties. Subsequently, the capacity to tolerate the child's sexual intrusions, competitiveness, and hostility during the oedipal phase tests the parental capacity to retain optimal distance. The child's diminished need of parents during latency and the intense, often maddening, oscillations in attitudes, affect, and distance during adolescence similarly require parental object constancy and solidity of identity if all is to go well.

Still later, middle age mobilizes a broadening of the core self-representation and a compensatory deepening of what one indeed has become. In his writings, Erikson (1950a, 1956) emphasized the new psychosocial level of integration of identity in later life.

Kernberg (1980) extended this theme to the internal world. According to him, in middle age

> one should be able to come to terms with the limits of change derived from one's character, one's personality structure, and with the related repetitive cycles of activation of one's internalized object relations, which are enacted, again and again, as a limited repertoire of "personal myths." . . . To accept oneself within such limits is an important aspect of emotional maturity that is in contrast to narcissistic rationalization, to denial, to resignation and cynicism, and to masochistic self blame. [p. 127]

Kohut (1977) also writes of late middle age as a time when we "ask ourselves whether we have been true to our innermost design" (p. 241). Self-scrutiny of this sort is inevitably associated with mourning for the self-representations that have remained mute and unexpressed in lived life. Sadness appears on the scene and the subjective awareness of passing time becomes acute. My 1992 poem, "Calendar" seeks to capture this very subterranean anguish of middle age.

> A page turns
> And suddenly what was love
>   is simply a "valuable experience" from the past.
> You stop pushing the outsides of the envelope,
>   stay within,
>   feel relieved that the polyp in your throat is benign,
>   can be removed easily.
> A page turns.
>   You need glasses to read.
>   Your son leaves for college.
> And, suddenly, fall is in the air.

Such "fall," however, is not devoid of ego benefits. Letting go of the children provides a greater opportunity for furthering intimacy with one's spouse and deepening one's commitment to work. Enhanced monetary security, more time for self-reflection, and greater ease of travel also offer opportunities for further ego growth and refinement of identity. The birth of grandchildren, in later middle age, is especially joyous in its offer of "genetic immortality" (Colarusso 1997, p. 91) and the illusion of possessing a self that will outlast time (see also Cath 1997). The deep emotional involvement with grandchildren serves multiple purposes. According to Colarusso (1997), these include their offering one: "(i) A narcissistic buffer against the stings of old age and the inevitability of death, (ii) a chance for magical repair of one's own life through genetic immortality, and (iii) a denial of unalterable imperfections in the self through selective identification with particular qualities in the grandchild" (pp. 90–91).

Finally, during old age and as one approaches death and is "on the way to second symbiosis" (Madow 1997), so to speak, a deep and post-ambivalent view of the world that one has lived in and is about to leave needs to be developed in order for this final transition to be smooth.

PHENOMENOLOGICAL ASPECTS

> The consciously available sense of identity is derived from the current self concept, while an abiding sense of identity over time is derived from supraordinate self schemas, which integrate various subordinate self concepts and personal roles for relating with others.
> [Moore and Fine 1990, p. 93]

> To maintain a sense of belonging and continuity, it is important to have exposure to familiar symbols: the dress, the language, the food, and the participation in rituals all reinforce a sense of identity.
> [Ramanajum 1997, p. 144]

Realistic Body Image

An individual's identity is deeply anchored in the sense of his or her corporeal existence. Freud's (1923) declaration that "the ego is first and foremost a bodily ego" (p. 26) speaks to this very point. Two years after Freud's statement, Schilder (1935) described the concept of body image—the psychic representation of the body—and emphasized that this image is in a continuous process of construction and reconstruction throughout life. Individuals with a stable body image are able to maintain enduring and realistic perceptions of their physical attributes. In Winnicott's (1960, p. 44) terms, they display a true "psychosomatic existence." They feel solidly grounded in their own bodies, readily "recognize" themselves in a mirror, and are capable of making reasonable estimates of their weight, appearance, and body size. They display ego resilience and are able to adapt to ordinary (balding, or pregnancy) and extraordinary (amputation, accidental disfigurement) alterations of their bodies (Abse 1966, Winnicott 1949).

Subjective Self-Sameness

A consolidated identity provides an individual with the intrapsychic experience of subjective self-sameness. In diverse social situations, such individuals act and feel in a manner that is true to themselves. They experience themselves as essentially one personality and inwardly maintain similar preferences across various circumstances (Erikson 1950a,b, 1956, 1958, 1962). While interacting with different age groups or with individuals with whom they have varying levels of intimacy, they can modulate their behavior without losing a core sense of inner sameness. To be sure, the degree of such contextual flexibility varies from culture to culture, but the fact is that all individuals occasionally resort to some degree of social falseness, although not to the extent of actually deluding themselves in this regard. In this connection, Winnicott's (1965) observation that in health the false self is "represented by the whole organization of the polite and mannered social attitude" (p. 143) is pertinent.

Consistent Attitudes and Behaviors

Individuals who have achieved a healthy identity demonstrate consistent attitudes and behaviors. They display a stable investment in personal values and ideologies, and a related ability to recognize, focus upon, and articulate what is meaningful. Such persons also possess a repertoire of behaviors that assumes congruous and predictable parameters. They can be shy or exhibitionistic but not both, greedy or ascetic but not both. Their political ideologies, aesthetic interests, and tastes in food or music remain unaltered regardless of context. Wishes to act in ways that deviate too much from the prevailing sense of self are repressed or consciously inhibited and discouraged, thus maintaining a sense of internal consistency. At the same time, it must be emphasized that a healthy identity does not imply a rigid, monolithic homogeneity (Eisnitz 1980, Pfeiffer 1974). Indeed, a normal, well-integrated, and well-functioning identity is comprised of many subsets of self-representations (Eisnitz 1980) that manifest themselves as given psychosocial needs dictate. Contextual fluidity[24] of this sort is, however, distinct from identity diffusion. What differentiates a cohesive identity from a poorly integrated one is the former's overall synthesis, comfortable transition between various self-representations, and optimal mixture of reality principle and ego ideal-dictated direction in manifesting or not manifesting various facets of oneself. The necklace of identity has many beads to be sure, but they are connected by a meaningful and adaptive thread.

Temporal Continuity

An essential characteristic of individuals with consolidated identity is their capacity to maintain personal continuity amid change and with the passing of time (Erikson 1950a, 1956, Lichtenstein 1963). Stern's (1985) concept of "self history," that is, a sense of enduring and of a continuation with one's own subjective past, refers to this specific capacity. Individuals who possess it retain genuine ties with their past, comfortably locate themselves in their current realities, and can envision their future. They maintain regular contact with people and places known and visited in the

---

24. That Indian and Pakistani individuals show great fluidity of identity has been noted by both Ewing (1991) and Roland (1996).

past, keep photographs and mementos from various life experiences, and write personal journals or in other ways carry on an ongoing synthesis of what is left behind with what is at hand. Sometimes such temporal synthesis requires actual visits to old places, old friends, parents, or even parental graves (Akhtar and Smolar 1998). At other times, mending of various time segments of life can only occur in fantasy and reverie. This is certainly more common in immigrants and is well depicted in the following lines of a poem by Darius Cooper (1995), an Indian–North American poet.

> As darkness falls,
> I look at my son's beautiful sleeping face,
> His tiny palms
> Firmly closed
> Over the weight of his world,
> And I think of my parents
> As they dream of holding him
> In their arms,
> In a small town
> Far far away. [p. 41]

Temporal fluidity prevents fixity of identity in one particular personal era, leaving open the possibility of transformations over the course of life (Akhtar 1984, Kernberg 1980, Levinson et al. 1978, Wolman and Thompson 1990). However, such transformations are cumulative and discrete, not grotesque (e.g., "midlife crisis") in nature. Ideally, development is like the growth of a tree. Rings accumulate around a central core without altering a shape that remains recognizable year after year. This paradox that individuals with a consolidated identity change so much and yet remain the same, as it were, is attributed by Emde (1983) to an ever-present affective continuity in the psychic life.

Authenticity

As a subject of psychological investigation, authenticity has acquired myriad definitions in Western psychological thought (Frankl 1959, Maslow 1971, Trilling 1968). *Merriam-Webster's New*

Collegiate Dictionary (1987) defines authentic as that which is "worthy of acceptance or belief, conforming to fact or reality, not imaginary or false" (p. 117). Following this definition, Webster's notes that authenticity involves being actually and exactly what is claimed; without counterfeit; being fully genuine, sincere and trustworthy.

From this perspective, individuals with a crystallized identity are authentic (Akhtar 1984, Kernberg 1975, 1976, Volkan 1976, Winnicott 1965). They are knowledgeable about and committed to an intrapsychic and interpersonal ideology that has as its credo the experience of being true toward oneself and others. As well as having a capacity for originality, such persons are able to recognize and accept the facts about themselves as they see them. Dietary preferences, selection of clothing, likes and dislikes of art, literature, or music, tastes in decorating one's home, and selection of leisure activities emanate from a deep and mostly unconscious synthesis of early identifications with one's own actual life experience. There is little effort at imitating others in these matters.[25]

Gender

Individuals with a consolidated identity possess a subjective clarity regarding their gender (Jacobson 1954, Mahler et al. 1975, Volkan 1976). Gender identity, one index of ego development, consists of three aspects that are essential for an integrated self-identity. These are: (1) core gender identity (Stoller 1968), or the awareness and acceptance of having one or the other type of genitals and therefore of being male or female; (2) gender role (Green 1975), or one's overt behavior in relationship to other people with respect to one's gender, and (3) sexual partner orientation, or one's preferred sex of the love object. A cohesive gender identity is concordant with one's biological sex and shows harmony between core gender identity, gender role, and sexual partner ori-

---

25. Focal areas of inauthenticity (e.g., in realms of attire or accent) in the early phases of immigration are common, and exist along with a deep capacity for genuineness in areas of life unaffected by migration.

entation. This translates into heterosexual object choice—a matter that has become increasingly controversial—and an overall demeanor societally considered gender consistent. Such solid gender identity emerges from the interplay of constitutional givens and cultural factors, with deep acceptance of the distinction between the sexes, the predominance of identifications with the same-sex parent, and a recognition of the complementarity of the opposite sex (Green 1975, Mahler et al. 1975, Stoller 1968).

Ethnicity and Conscience

Ethnicity refers to the culture of a people and includes values, child-rearing practices, sense of history, modes of expression, and patterns of interpersonal behavior (Hughes 1993). Ethnicity is transmitted to children by exposure to the family's cultural mores and by the ethnic "language" within the family. Through identifications with parents, especially during the oedipal phase, the child gradually acquires a sense of generational continuity (Chasseguet-Smirgel 1984). Extension of this sense results in a feeling of belonging to an historical community. In Volkan's (1988) words, "By identifying with others in one's own group—parental figures, peer groups, teachers, religious authorities, community and national leaders—one identifies with their investment in religion, ethnicity, nationality, and so on, and shares in the differentiation of those persons unlike the group and inimical to it" (p. 49).

Such ethnic identity is "both positive (*we do this*) and negative (*we do not do what they do*)" (Thomson et al. 1993, original italics). This early ethnic sense, which may border on ethnocentricity, gets diluted during adolescence when a certain disidentification with parental mores occurs (Blos 1967, Jacobson 1954, Money and Ehrhardt 1972). The wider interaction with diverse social and ethnic groups that takes place at this time facilitates a diminution of childhood ethnocentricity. However, ethnicity survives past adolescence and imparts a sense of historical depth to the adult identity.

Behaviorally, this translates into an awareness (if not active observance) of religious festivals, a subtle preference for homoethnic ties, a fondness for certain foods and music, and the use of linguistic expressions consistent with one's ethnic roots. A related phenomenon is that persons with healthy identities demonstrate an internalized value system. Ideals and personal convictions are constant over time, and there is no real vulnerability to be manipulated by demagogues or esoteric sects.

CLINICAL RELEVANCE

> Identity is a coherent sense of self. It depends upon the awareness that one's endeavors and one's life make sense, that they are meaningful in the context in which life is lived. It depends also upon stable values, and upon the conviction that one's actions and values are harmoniously related. [Wheelis 1958, p. 19]

> . . . identity diffusion is reflected in a history of grossly contradictory behavior, or in an alteration between emotional states implying such grossly contradictory behavior and perception of the self that the interviewer finds it very difficult to see the patient as a "whole" human being. [Kernberg 1984, p. 13]

Recognition of what constitutes a well-consolidated identity is relevant for all three aspects of patient care in clinical psychiatry: differential diagnosis, treatment, and estimation of prognosis. In the diagnostic realm, it is safe to assume that the greater the identity disturbance the more severe is the underlying psychopathology. Indeed, disorders of identity seem to exist on the following continuum of increasing severity: (1) *identity crisis*, which is a transient upheaval in the sense of an individual's identity during adolescence; (2) *identity diffusion*, which involves disturbances of the seven assets of identity described above and is typical of borderline, narcissistic, schizoid, hypomanic, antisocial, paranoid, as-if, and schizotypal personalities (Akhtar 1984, 1992b, Akhtar and Samuel 1996, Erikson 1956, 1958, Grinker, et al. 1968, Kernberg 1970, 1975); (3) *identity dissociation*, which involves the amnestically sequestered existence of personified self-representations and is typical of multiple personality (Akhtar 1984, Janet 1907, Prince 1905); and (4) *identity fragmentation,* which refers to the bizarre transformations of the self, a breakdown of the boundaries of one's identity, and is characteristic of psychotic decompensation (Akhtar and Brown 1999, Batchelor 1969, Bleuler 1908, Diefendorf 1921, Fish 1964, Hinsie and Campbell 1975, Slater and Roth 1969).

Because the gross forms of identity disturbance (e.g., fragmentation, dissociation) are often readily discernible, the importance of the concept of identity mainly resides in its usefulness when distinguishing "higher level" or neurotic type (e.g., avoidant, obsessional) personality disorders from "lower level" or severe (e.g., borderline, antisocial, paranoid, schizoid) personality disorders (Kernberg 1970). Individuals of the former type possess a cohesive identity, whereas individuals of the latter type suffer from the "syndrome of identity diffusion" (Akhtar 1984, 1992b, Erikson 1956, 1958, Grinker, et al. 1968, Kernberg 1970, 1975). They display defects in the seven aspects of identity described above. However the degree to which identity diffusion is readily manifest varies greatly. For instance, borderline individuals display these phenomena more overtly than narcissistic patients, who are better integrated. Also, the various manifestations of identity diffusion do not occur to an equal degree in all patients with identity diffusion. Narcissistic patients may display more inauthenticity, borderline patients more temporal discontinuity, and schizotypal patients more feelings of emptiness, for instance. Such clinical impressions, if operationalized and replicated, might help in developing better phenomenological profiles of these conditions.

The concepts of identity and identity diffusion have treatment implications as well. Individuals with consolidated identities require different therapeutic strategies when compared to their counterparts with identity diffusion. Psychoanalysis, which explores unconscious dynamics, defensive operations, and transference manifestations in a setting of ego regression, is appropriate only for individuals with consolidated identities (Akhtar 1992b, Bachrach and Leaff 1978). There are three reasons for this. *First,* individuals with a consolidated identity have a capacity for relating to others as separate and autonomous objects. This capacity facilitates their developing and sustaining a "therapeutic" (Greenson 1965) or "working" (Brenner 1979) alliance with the analyst, a requirement essential for the observation of transference fantasies and affects with a certain detachment. Transference-based misconceptions and emotional storms can thus become (and remain) amenable to scrutiny and understanding. *Second,* since "predominance of love is the glue of the unified representation" (Settlage 1991, p. 352), individuals with a consolidated identity, by definition, bring more love than hate with them to a clinical situation. The amount of aggression associated with their conflicts is manageable within the confines of a verbal dialogue and within the illusory nature of re- lationship inherent to psychoanalysis. In other words, hate only minimally propels them toward hostile and dangerous actions and can therefore be contained in the analytic dialogue without the analyst having to depart from neutrality. *Third,* since a consolidated identity implies a better integrated character and a greater capac- ity to utilize insight-oriented interventions, it is also an indicator for favorable outcome of psychotherapy and psychoanalysis.

Individuals with identity diffusion, in contrast, lack the solid core of self-experience necessary for a regressive and potentially desta- bilizing treatment such as psychoanalysis. Even the ones in this group who are amenable to and motivated for a deep and sustained modification of their lives require some combination of insight- oriented and supportive measures. Many approaches to their treat- ment exist, as is evident from the enormous growth of literature on this subject over the last two or three decades. Among the views represented here are those based on object relations theory (Kernberg 1975, 1976, 1984, Volkan 1976, 1987), Kleinian metapsychology (Grotstein 1981, Rosenfeld 1987), views of the independent group of British psychoanalysts (Balint 1968, Guntrip 1969, Khan 1974, 1983), and their exponents in this country (Adler 1985, Lewin and Schulz 1992, Modell 1984), therapeutic ap- proaches evolving from the impact of the interpersonal tradition on mainstream psychoanalysis (Searles 1986) and from certain specific developmental paradigms (Masterson 1976, Rinsley 1982), self-psychology (Kohut 1977), and other mixed theoretical viewpoints (Boyer and Giovacchini 1980, Gunderson 1985). While these viewpoints emphasize different nuances of therapeutic technique, they do seem to hold a consensus that psychoanalysis, in its unmodified form, is not the treatment of choice for individuals with identity diffusion. With this proviso, the therapeutic approaches emanating from the diverse theoretical viewpoints outlined above can broadly be seen as belonging to two different camps. One camp (Adler 1985, Balint 1968, Guntrip 1969, Khan 1974, 1983, Kohut 1977, Lewin and Schulz 1992, Modell 1984) emphasizes "affirmative interventions" (Killingmo 1989) that provide holding, mirroring, and containing to the patient's tormented self experience in an effort to facilitate resumption of thwarted development that underlies the patient's malady. The other camp (Grotstein 1981, Kernberg 1975, 1976, 1984, Rosenfeld 1987, Searles 1986, Volkan 1976, 1987) underscores the need for unmasking the unconscious reasons for the patient's mental compartmentalization and of "bridging interventions" (Akhtar 1995b, 1998a) aimed at mending contradictions by pointing them out and thus creating a capacity for ambivalence toward self and others. Hybrid approaches (Akhtar 1992b, 1999d, Killingmo 1989, Modell 1984) also exist and most clinicians perhaps intuitively attempt to strike their own variety of balance between these two positions.

In light of its multifaceted relevance, identity warrants assessment in the clinical situation.[26] However, not all facets of identity can be explored and not all features of identity diffusion can be elicited to an equal degree through formal questioning during the clinical interview. Some of the latter (e.g., feelings of emptiness) are more evident in the patient's complaints, while others (e.g., temporal discontinuity in the self-experience) become clear only through obtaining a longitudinal account of the patient's life. Still other features (e.g., subtle disturbances of gender identity) are discernible, at least in the beginning, mainly through the overall manner of the patient's relating to the interviewer. Yet it is almost

---

26. For an up-to-date summary of psychometric inventories for assessing identity consolidation, see Akhtar and Samuel (1996).

always helpful to ask the patient to describe himself or herself (Akhtar 1992b, Kernberg 1984). Of course, such an inquiry begins only after the patient's presenting symptomatology has been discussed. At this point, the interviewer might say something like this: "Well, now that you have told me about your difficulties and we have talked about them for a while, can you please describe yourself as a person?" In the description offered, one should look for consistency versus contradiction, clarity versus confusion, solidity versus emptiness, well-developed and comfortably experienced masculinity or femininity versus gender confusion, and a sense of inner morality and ethnicity versus the lack of any historical or communal anchor.

However, if the patient is unable to provide a coherent self-description, this should not be automatically construed as showing identity diffusion, as it could be due to anxiety, lack of psychological-mindedness, cultural factors, poor verbal skills, or low intelligence. These factors should be ruled out before making a conclusion regarding the presence or absence of identity diffusion. Moreover, a less than forthcoming patient is often helped in this regard by a piecemeal inquiry. For instance, the interviewer might ask about the patient's religious beliefs, practices, and their continuity with what was handed down to him during childhood; feelings of ethnicity and of belonging to a certain regional or communal group; continuity with friends and associates from earlier periods of life; clarity and stability of vocational goals; sublimations and hobbies; legal record; drug use and drinking, and so on. He may then make a surmise about the patient's identity based on the information gathered. A patient might not be able to describe himself well, yet may turn out to possess a consolidated identity. Conversely, one might come across in a patient

> peripheral areas of self-experience that are contradictory to a well-integrated, central area of subjective experience, peripheral areas that the patient experiences as ego-alien or ego-dystonic, not fitting into his otherwise integrated picture of himself. These isolated areas may be an important source of intrapsychic conflict or interpersonal difficulties but should not be equated with identity diffusion. [Kernberg 1984, p. 37]

In the case of immigrant patients, the assessment of identity-related issues, while not eclipsing their other complaints, is of paramount importance. Initial interviews with such patients must pay attention to the reasons the individuals have arrived in a new country and the extent and manner of their adaptation to this profound change. Ignoring this important area of the patient's psyche, at times in an unconscious collusion with the patient's own narcissism-based denial of his immigrant status (Smolar 1999), can lead to subsequent blind spots during the treatment.[27]

SUMMARY

> The process of American identity formation seems to support an individual's ego identity as long as he can preserve a certain element of deliberate tentativeness of autonomous choice. The individual must be able to convince himself that the next step is up to him and that no matter where he is staying or going he always has the choice of leaving or turning in the opposite direction if he chooses to do so. [Erikson 1950, p. 286]

This chapter has synthesized the scattered psychiatric and psychoanalytic literature on the topic and shed light on the historical origins, development, phenomenology, and clinical relevance of identity. Results of this synthesis reveal the following: (1) The concept of identity has persisted over eight decades. (2) Identity emanates within the earliest interplay of the infant's temperament with the maternal attitude, gains structure from primitive introjections, refines itself through later selective identifications, acquires filiation and generational continuity in passage through the Oedipus complex, and arrives at its more or less final shape through syn-

---

27. I am struck by the number of immigrant colleagues who have told me that little attention was paid to their immigrant status during their otherwise satisfactory analyses!

thesis of contradictory identifications and greater individuation during adolescence, though this too remains subject to further refinements through young adulthood, midlife, and even old age. (3) A cohesive identity is composed of a realistic body image, subjective self-sameness, consistent attitudes, temporality, gender clarity, authenticity, and ethnicity. (4) Disturbance of identity suggests psychopathology with greater identity disturbance being associated with progressively more severe conditions, such as severe personality disorders, multiple personality, or psychosis. (5) Clinical assessment is therefore relevant and might indicate treatment strategies and outcome expectations. The need for such assessment is increased manyfold in the immigrant, who is almost invariably struggling with various threats to his identity.

3

FOUR TRACKS
IN IDENTITY
TRANSFORMATION
FOLLOWING
IMMIGRATION

Regardless of whether it is from one country to another or from one region to another region of the same country, immigration always causes a certain "culture shock" (Garza-Guerrero 1974, Handlin 1973, Ticho 1971). The consequent anxiety challenges the stability of the newcomer's psychic organization. Another threat is posed by the mourning over the losses inherent in immigration. This coexistence of culture shock and mourning causes a serious shake-up of the individual's identity. A state of psychic flux ensues and

> a growing sensation of discontinuity of identity emerges. It is as if, out of his usual habitat, the newcomer no longer has the necessary corroborative environmental feedback for his ego identity. . . . The severity of the threats to the individual identity runs parallel to the severity of concomitant mourning. Thus, the more serious the break with the newcomer's continuity of his identity, the greater his yearning for those lost love objects (abandoned culture) which in the past provided a comfortable sense of continuity. On the other hand, the greater his longing for those lost love objects, the more afflictive the threats to his identity. [Garza-Guerrero 1974, pp. 418–419]

This intrapsychic turmoil is reminiscent of the "second individuation process of adolescence" (Blos 1967). Reaching ontogenetically backwards, one can also discern psychodynamic echoes of the childhood separation-individuation phase (Mahler et al. 1975)—the first stepping-stone for identity formation—in the immigrant's turmoil. However, such phenomenological resemblance does not mean genetic equation. Individuals migrating at significantly later stages of development undergo characterologic processes that are certainly more subtle and complex than those of early childhood or even adolescence. Much psychic structuralization has already ensued in these individuals; drives have attained fusion and genital primacy, ego is better organized, and a post-adolescence superego is in place. Their moral, aesthetic, social temporal, and linguistic transformation as a result of immigration is more a matter of adult adaptation than of a replicated childhood scenario, though the two cannot be entirely separated.

It is against such a backdrop that the following four interconnected tracks of identity change upon immigration should be considered. These tracks (and the associated metaphoric journeys) involve the dimensions of drives and affects (from love or hate to ambivalence), interpersonal and psychic space (from near or far to optimal distance), temporality (from yesterday or tomorrow to today), and social affiliations and mutuality (from yours or mine to ours). To be sure, there are caveats and pitfalls in such conceptualizations, but I will address them after describing the four tracks in some detail.

FROM LOVE OR HATE TO AMBIVALENCE

> Idealized, "all good" object images have to be integrated with "all bad" object images, and the same holds true for good and bad self images. In this process of synthesis, partial images of the self and of the objects are integrated into total object and self representations, and thus self and object representations become . . . more realistic. [Kernberg 1975, p. 27]

> It is possible that we move beyond splitting by flickering back and forth fast enough to begin to see new pictures, much as the illusion of motion in motion

> pictures depends upon a succession of still pictures
> rapid enough to enlist persistence of vision to pro-
> duce the subjective experience of continuity. [Lewin
> and Schulz 1992, p. 51]

Like the rapprochement subphase toddler (Mahler et al. 1975) and the transiently regressed adolescent (Blos 1967, Kramer 1980), the immigrant is vulnerable to splitting of self- and object representations (Kernberg 1967) along libidinal and aggressive lines. The drastic change in his external environment taxes the ego's adaptive capacities. Changed societal dictates on acceptable behavior cause drive disregulation. A male immigrant from a sexually repressive culture such as Saudi Arabia or Iraq might find the casual friendliness of Western women uncomfortably stimu-lating. A female from a similar background might unconsciously equate the Western woman with the oedipal rival and be stirred in her aggressive and competitive strivings. Or, on the other hand, the day-to-day intermingling with men might stimulate her re-pressed erotic longings. In contrast to this, a Western immigrant to a culture such as Japan, which prizes group affiliation over individuation, might be suddenly faced with his repudiated sym-biotic longings and wishes for masochistic submission to a disso-ciated harsh superego. Regardless of the specific form it takes, the cultural change consequent upon immigration is bound to test ego resilience both from the outside and from the forces unleashed within.

An early consequence is the phenomenon of "disorienting anxi-ety" (Grinberg and Grinberg 1989), which arises from

> problems in differentiating one's feelings about two subjects of in-
> terest and conflict: the country and people one has left behind
> and the new environment. . . . The emigrant experiences this as
> if his parents were divorced, and he engages in fantasies of form-
> ing an alliance with one against the other. Confusion increases
> when culture, language, place, points of reference, memories, and
> experiences become mixed up and superimposed on one another.
> Confused states also result from defensive attempts to stave off per-
> secutory anxieties in the face of the unknown. [pp. 87–88]

Before more adaptive ego defenses can be put into place, regression is a mechanism frequently resorted to.[28] Splitting becomes predominant and colors the immigrant's feelings about his two lands and his own two self-representations. The country of origin is idealized, the new culture devalued. For an East-to-West immigrant, this often gives rise to the idea that Western culture is characterized by greed, sexual promiscuity, violence, and disregard of generational boundaries, while the Eastern culture is seen as a place of contentment, instinctual restraint, love, humility, and respect for the young and the old. For an immigrant who goes from the West to East, a similar splitting of object representations yields a view of the East as riddled with indolence, filth, superstition, subservience, and pathetic withering of instincts, while the West is viewed as industrious, conscientious, orderly, instinctually gratifying, and encouraging of self-actualization.

Four things need to be added here. *First,* these split views are subject to shifts; the resulting change in emotion leads to a sense of conviction about one's altered views. One day the country of origin is idealized and the country of adoption is devalued. Next day, it is the reverse. *Second,* while they are phenomenologically akin to the splitting of the rapprochement subphase, such contradictory attitudes contain the projective repudiation of developmentally higher-level conflicts as well. Falk (1974), for instance, has noted that countries or territories on the two sides of a border often unconsciously symbolize early parental figures. One country (usually that of origin) might come to represent mother, and the other country, father, thus setting up a fertile ground for oedipal fantasy and enactment on the immigrant's part. *Third,* and not restricted to the object world, splitting also afflicts the immigrant's self-representation. Being Belgian, Brazilian, Chinese, German,

---

28. A practicing subphase like hypomania is also characteristic of this early period of entry into a new culture. It has both defensive and adaptive functions. However, unlike the early anxieties, this hypomania is never fully renounced. It resurfaces again and again throughout the remaining life cycle whenever the need for mastering new cultural tasks arises (Anni Bergman, personal communication, April 1994).

Indian, Iranian, Korean, or Filipino tends to be libidinized, and to become a source of pride. The newly emergent self-representation, say American, is devalued and seems shameful. Indeed, such one-sided instinctual investment often reverses itself; what was once idealized becomes devalued and vice-versa. Here also, the phenomenological similarity with childhood libidinal-aggressive splitting should not lead one to overlook other (e.g., bisexual, oedipal) issues that might be involved. For instance, one self-representation might become imbued with male and the other with female attributes,[29] one with the oedipally accepting and the other with oedipally defiant qualities in the unconscious. In this connection, it is fascinating to note that while all continents have feminine names (Falk 1974), countries can exist as male or female in the unconscious. Awad (personal communication, 1995) for instance, notes that

> some Arab countries are female, while others are male. For example, Egypt, Palestine, and Syria are female, and when you talk about a "beloved country," the feminine verb *Habiba* appears as in *Misr* (Egypt) *Al-Habiba*. On the other hand, Lebanon, Jordan, and Iraq are male, and the verbs associated with them are masculine verbs, such as *Lubnan Al-Habib*.

Finally, if pre-existing vulnerabilities of character come together with inordinate frustrations emanating from external realities, aggression spills into all significant object relations. Under such circumstances, the immigrant feels hatred not only for his country of adoption but also for his country of origin. A regressive anger of this sort is displayed in the terse language of my 1979 poem "Two Homes" about immigration.[30]

---

29. Silber (1994) has recently argued that around the end of the Civil War the North constructed a feminized interpretation of the South which validated the former's superiority. In emphasizing Southern helplessness, the Northerners even couched descriptions of Southern landscapes in feminine terms.

30. The cynical tone, the taut construction, and the contemptuous devaluation of both countries (India and the United States) is obvious here. However,

> From the land of sounds to the land of colors
> is a long distance
> From the waste of appetite to the waste of food
> is a long distance
> From the shame of begging to the horror of mugging
> is a long distance
> From the termites of stoicism to the tyranny of pursuit
> is a long distance
> From the asepsis of asceticism to the squalor of
> indulgence
> is a long distance
> From the greed of worship to the worship of greed
> is a long distance
> and
> From the home of my boyhood to the home of my boy's
> boyhood
> is a long distance

Hatred for either the new or the old country is frequently a defense against guilt. This mechanism was pointed out long ago by Jones (1928), who noted that

> Hatred for someone implies that the other person, through his cruelty or unkindness, is the cause of one's sufferings, that the latter are not self-imposed or in any way one's own fault. All the responsibility for the misery produced by unconscious guilt is thus displaced onto the other, supposedly cruel person, who is therefore heartily hated. [p. 384]

---

in attempting to understand this poem twenty years after it was written, I begin to see something more in it. The reassuring and rhythmic repetition of "is a long distance" now begins to appear as a literary "inconstant object" (Blum 1981) par excellence; in other words, the repetition, even though of seemingly aggressive words, contains soothing and libidinal aspects as well. Toward the end of the poem, the wistful idealization of our (mine and my son's) "boyhood" also provides hope for libido's predominance over aggression, and of love winning out over hate. Seen through this altered prism, the repeated phrase "long distance" no longer remains a reminder of the gap between two lands but also an unconscious allusion to "long distance" phone calls that can bring the two lands together!

In the case of an immigrant, there are many sources of unconscious guilt. These include guilt at success in the new country
(standing for an incestuous triumph), "separation guilt" (Modell
1965) from the old country, and "survivor's guilt" (Niederland
1968) in general. Such guilt, as stated in Chapter 1, is likely to be
greater in those emigrating from socioeconomically disadvantaged
and politically unstable regions.

Gradually, a synthesis of two self representations sets in. For this
to take place, however, ample sustenance of "growth needs" (Casement 1991, p. 274), enough "efficacy experiences" (Wolf 1994, p.
73), and a positive balance of libido over aggression are necessary.
Settlage's (1992) succinct remark, made in connection with the
initial achievement of self-constancy, is no less pertinent here: "The
predominance of love is the glue of a unified self-representation"
(p. 352). As a result of this synthesis, capacity for good-humored
ambivalence toward both the country of origin and that of adoption develops. A hyphenated identity now emerges. Such an identity might lack deep historical anchoring in either of the historical and identification systems but might possess a greater than usual
breadth of experience—a sense of relativity, knowledge, and, at
times, wisdom. An external manifestation of this psychostructural
achievement is the immigrant's increasing comfort in simultaneously associating with individuals from his two cultures. A
"mixed" guest list for a dinner at the immigrant's house is a tell-
tale sign of such advance in identity consolidation.

FROM NEAR OR FAR TO OPTIMAL DISTANCE

> Going away leads to different consequences for a
> man's human and non-human experience. He can
> reproduce the old life with people in the new place,
> because people do not differ greatly from one to the
> other. He eventually finds new friends. But places
> can differ so profoundly that it is no longer possible
> to have certain sorts of experiences of place at all.
> Such deprivations and losses inevitably increase
> awareness of the non-human world, both the old and
> the new. [Denford 1981, p. 325]

> It was not simply owing to the stressful circumstances
> attending the emigration that I became newly cre-
> ative. It was rather that, with the stress came new vis-
> tas, new curiosity, new opportunities, and vital new
> sources of collegiate support. It was only in America,
> and only owing to the tremendous professional en-
> couragement I received in America, that I no longer
> felt I was laboring under the shadow of titans. [Mar-
> garet Mahler, in Stepansky 1988, p. 121]

Elsewhere, I have reviewed in detail the conceptual ambiguities, developmental origins, cultural vicissitudes, and technical implications of optimal distance (Akhtar 1992a). Here it will suffice to say that it is a hybrid concept (Balint 1959, Bouvet 1958, Escoll 1992) that can be viewed from both interpersonal and intrapsychic perspectives. Mahler herself (Mahler et al. 1975) describes it as both a position "between mother and child that best allows the infant to develop those faculties which he needs in order to grow, that is, to individuate" (p. 291), and as a later ego capacity for establishing an optimal distance from the internal representation of the mother (and subsequently of others). She notes that during the symbiotic phase, there is no outside world for the infant, no distance. Gradually, there develops "the space between mother and child" (Bergman 1980, p. 201). Created both by the mother's comings and goings and by a decrease in the baby's bodily dependence upon her, this space[31] permits the child to look "beyond the symbiotic orbit" (Mahler 1974, p. 155). The infant attempts to break away from the passive lap-babyhood. During the practicing subphase, the child shows even greater ability to move away from the mother, at first by crawling and later by upright locomotion. The child makes pleasurable forays in the external world and seems oblivious to the mother's presence. Yet, revealing his continued need for a home base, he periodically returns to the mother. In the rapprochement subphase, no distance from the mother ap-

---

31. Winnicott (1971) is also interested in this space. However, his focus is not upon the child's ambivalent efforts to minimize it but upon its persistence and varying psychic uses throughout life.

pears satisfactory, but if the mother remains emotionally available despite the child's oscillations the capacity for optimal distance gradually develops.

Reverberations of these themes can be found in the immigrant's interpersonal and intrapsychic life. At the external level, the immigrant has to rediscover the acceptable limits of interpersonal space (see Hall [1973] and Zerubavel [1991] for a sociological perspective on interpersonal distance). The extent of physical contact, spatial proximity, and psychological intimacy becomes a matter of renewed psychosocial negotiation and practice. More importantly, the immigrant finds himself "too far" from his country of origin, a distance that he, like the practicing-phase toddler, might greatly enjoy for some time. Sooner or later, however, the anxiety of having exceeded the symbiotic orbit surfaces. The immigrant's ego loses the support it had drawn from the familiar environment, climate, and landscape—all unconsciously perceived as extensions of the mother (Krystal and Petty 1963). "Attempts at restoration of such ego support may lead the immigrant to seek a climate and ethnic surrounding much like his original, and [he] may become involved in a life-long attempt at symbolic restitution of his motherland" (Krystal 1966, p. 217).[32] A fantasy of return to the home country also emerges. The wish, like the rapprochement-subphase child's regressive search for symbiosis, is, however, not free of ambivalence. In myriad rationalized ways, acting upon it is postponed. Conditions (e.g., saving money, earning a diploma) are set for one's return but their fulfillment eludes the immigrant like a mirage.[33] The poignancy of one's being on such an existential treadmill is well-captured by the London-based Urdu poet, Iftikhar Aarif.

---

32. According to Krystal (1966), the artist Giorgio de Chirico's preoccupation with Italian landscapes is a conspicuous example of such a need.

33. It is not uncommon for immigrants to wish to be buried, after their deaths, in their homelands. The fantasy of return thus remains alive in them. In this connection, it is interesting to note that some eight years before her death, Margaret Mahler had arranged to have her ashes transported to Sopron, Hungary, and interred in the Jewish cemetery next to her father's grave (Stepansky 1988).

Azaab yeh bhi kisi aur par nahin aaya.
Tamaam umr chaley aur ghar nahin aaya.

[There are few who have been so cursed
To wander all one's life and never arrive at home.] [Aarif 1983, p. 87]

A frequent stopgap measure in this ongoing agony is actual travel
back to the country of origin. Carrying gifts to the relatives left
behind, and bringing back cultural artifacts and mementos upon
return to his new home, the immigrant reminds one of a toddler
crisscrossing the space between himself and his mother. Bergman's
(1980) comment, though made in the latter connection, seems
equally applicable to the immigrant.

> As . . . he is able to move away farther, his world begins to widen,
> there is more to see, more to hear, more to touch, and each time
> he returns to mother he brings with him some of the new experi-
> ence. In other words, each time he returns he is ever so slightly
> changed. The mother is the center of his universe to whom he re-
> turns as the circles of his exploration widen. [p. 203]

The distance between two lands (two mothers, the "mother of
symbiosis" and the "mother of separation") is also bridged by
homoethnic ties in the new country, international phone calls, and
listening to one's native music.[34] These serve as "transitional objects" (Winnicott 1953) and help bring what has become externally
"too far" a bit nearer. A related concept is that of "transitional

---

34. A poignant ritual that embodied the psychological "tether" fantasy
(Akhtar 1992b) was practiced by Italian women immigrants during the late nine-
teenth century. As their boats took off from the shores of Italy, they would hold
onto a ball of yarn, the other end of which was in the hands of friends remaining back. With the boat moving on forward, they would let the ball unravel with
the yarn still connecting them to their friends. Sooner or later, however, the
yarn would come to an end, become taut, and then break. The disconnected
yarn would now be floating on water, an anguished and resigned reminder of
their internal connection to their motherland (Dominic Mazza, personal communication 1999).

actions," described specifically in connection with exiles and refugees by Groenenberg (1999). These refer to

> sorts of rituals by means of which people try to bridge the distance between the reality and the ideal. Political demonstrations on a remembrance day, for example, form a link with the homeland and provide the opportunity for refugees to make their ideology known, to share their anger with others, and most important, to experience solidarity. In addition, music, film or theatre in which injustice in the homeland is denounced fulfill a similar function. These actions mark their ethnic identity, connect them to their own country and distinguish them from the people of the new country. At the same time, there is a communicative aspect in it towards the new country.

On an internal level too, the immigrant fluctuates between extremes of distance from his native self-representation and his newly emerging self representation as a resident of the adopted country. Failure to negotiate the distance between these self representations results in two problematic outcomes of identity (Teja and Akhtar 1981): ethnocentric withdrawal and counterphobic assimilation. Ethnocentric withdrawal involves clinging to an idealized view of one's earlier culture. Such individuals eat only their ethnic food and associate only with homoethnic groups.[35] Their residences, replete with artifacts from "back home," take on a shrine-like quality. They become more nationalistic toward their country of origin than they were while living in it. To buttress such secondary nationalism, they often forge unlikely alliances and develop new prejudices. Counterphobic assimilation is, in contrast, a caricature of the practicing subphase toddler. Intoxicated by the widening

---

35. Entire subcommunities (e.g., Chinatown, "Little Italy," the "Little Saigon" in Los Angeles, the Russian-Jewish community's "Odessa by the Sea" in New York's Brighton Beach area, the Indian communities in Edison, New Jersey, or Jackson Heights, Queens, New York) may have emerged on the basis of such ethnocentric withdrawal. These communities can serve as a refueling base for relatively more assimilated immigrants who do not live there but like to make frequent visits to such places.

horizons of their experiential world, these individuals totally renounce their original culture. In an "as-if" (Deutsch 1942) and "magic identification" (Jacobson 1964), they rapidly incorporate the host culture. Clearly, both ethnocentric withdrawal and counterphobic assimilation are multiply determined (Waelder 1936), although difficulty with aggression perhaps plays a large role here. More common are other solutions that appear to be compromise formations but nonetheless emanate from splitting of the self and object world. These include (1) pragmatic assimilation, which masks nonassimilation, the relationship between the two structures being akin to the "false" and "true" selves of Winnicott (1960); and (2) temporally alternating phases of closeness and distance from one or the other culture. The former individual lives a life that is assimilated from 9:00 a.m. to 5:00 p.m. and ethnocentric from 5:00 p.m. to 9:00 a.m. The latter goes through "native phases" and "assimilated phases" over a psychically undulating life. Both end up with a "life lived in pieces" (Pfeiffer 1974).

A deeper mending of being "too close" or "too far" from one or the other culture begins if the "holding environment" (Winnicott 1960), both within the family[36] and the culture at large, provides ample libidinal sustenance and containment of aggression. Manifestations of such mending include (1) increased comfort with one's ethnic or national origins at the workplace, along with a greater utilization of one's new self representation at home; this results in an enhanced "continuity of personal character" (Erikson 1956, p. 102), a hallmark of solid identity; (2) establishment of a predictable and reality-governed rhythm of refueling through international phone calls and visits; and (3) in the case of those who become parents in the adopted country, deeper acceptance of their offsprings' mixed but predominantly local loyalties.

---

36. In a study of 385 Soviet immigrant physicians to Israel, Ritsner and colleagues (1993) found the prevalence of depression to be strongly correlated with disturbed intrafamilial relations.

FROM YESTERDAY OR TOMORROW TO TODAY

> The failure of mourning leads to a continuing search
> for the idealized lost object, and inability to love new
> objects, a depreciation of objects in one's current
> life, and an endless pursuit of nostalgic memories for
> themselves at the expense of an inhibition in many
> areas of existence. [Werman 1977, p. 396]

> I would give all the landscapes of the world for that
> of my childhood. I must add, though, that if I make
> a paradise out of it, only the tricks or infirmity of
> memory can be held responsible. [E. M. Cioran 1982,
> p. 12, quoted in Amati-Mehler et al. 1993, p. 266]

The separation-individuation phase contains elements of mourning. With each progressive move toward autonomy and identity consolidation, there is an incremental loss of infantile omnipotence, symbiotic bliss, and ego simplification through splitting and projection. Compensation for this is found in the secondary narcissism of burgeoning ego capacities, autonomous functioning, a realistic self concept, and deeper object relations. Klein (1948), Winnicott (1953), and Mahler (1972) all trace a developmental line from illusion to disillusion during childhood. In Kleinian terms, this is a move from the "paranoid" to the depressive position. In the paranoid position, "goodness" is claimed for oneself and "badness" is totally externalized. The world is viewed in black-and-white terms. The self is regarded as an innocent victim and the other as an oppressor. Mistrust, fear, rage, greed, and ruthlessness predominate. In the depressive position, it is acknowledged that the self is not "all good" and the other not "all bad." The capacity for empathy appears on the horizon. There also emerge feelings of gratitude for what one has indeed received, guilt and sadness for having hurt others, and reparative longings to redress the damage done. Reality testing improves and the capacity for reciprocal relationships develops.

In Winnicott's (1953) terminology, initially "omnipotence is nearly a fact of life" (p. 238). Later, the transitional object appears, when the mother is in transition from being "merged with the infant to . . . being perceived rather than conceived of" (Winnicott 1971, p. 115). In Mahler's (Mahler et al. 1975) terminology, it is during the rapprochement subphase that the child realizes that his wishes and those of the mother do not always coincide. Unable to sustain the magic of symbiosis, "the child can no longer maintain his delusion of parental omnipotence" and also "must gradually and painfully give up the delusion of his own grandeur" (p. 79). Adding a significant nuance to Freud's (1911) outlining of the gradual replacement of pleasure principle by reality principle, Klein, Winnicott, and Mahler regard this journey from illusion to disillusion as necessary for psychic growth. A similar loss–restoration sequence is evident in the immigrant's psychic journey described so far. I will now focus upon the impact of it on his rootedness in the time experience.

Facing the "psychic pain" (Freud 1926b, p. 169) of separation, the immigrant often resorts to a hypercathexis of the lost objects. Described originally by Freud (1917) in "Mourning and Melancholia," this mechanism results in an idealization of the immigrant's past. Often such idealization centers more upon memories of places than of people. This is not surprising. Throughout childhood and adolescence, the nonhuman environment presents itself as a relatively neutral alternative area in which all the vicissitudes of human interactions can be expressed, experienced, and worked through in relative psychic privacy (Searles 1960). The inherent repudiation of aggression and the screen functions of nostalgia for lost places (Freedman 1956, Sterba 1940, Werman 1977) notwithstanding, the immigrant employing this mechanism comes to live in the past. Using Beiser's (1980) concepts of "time binding" (connectedness between the past, present, and future) and "time dominance" (the relative importance of each of these eras), one can say that for the immigrant time binding is disrupted and the past continues to exert time dominance. His most powerful affects are reserved for recall of the houses, street corners, cafes, hills, and countryside of his land. Like an emotionally deprived child with but one toy, the immigrant clings to memories. Ever wistful, he convinces himself that "if only" (Akhtar 1991, 1996) he had not left these places, his life would have been wonderful—or,

more frequently, that when he was there he had no problems. The
sharp retort of the great Urdu poet Ghalib (1841), finds no resonance in him. Ghalib said:

> Karte kis munh sey ho ghurbat ki shikayat Ghalib?
> Tum ko bemehriye—yaaran—e—watan yaad nahin?

> [O Ghalib, with what audacity do you complain of being in a strange
>   land?
> Have you forgotten the callousness of friends at home?] [p. 84]

Ghalib's reminder of prior frustrations is, on the other hand,
taken to heart by the individual who has had to leave his land
against his will or who was escaping from natural danger and/or
political persecution. Such a person feels differently cynical about
his country of origin. No wonder, since his internal experience is
strikingly different from the ordinary immigrant. Having to leave
against his will burdens him with a shameful experience of passiv-
ity and rejection. The suddenness of his departure deprives him
of the "protective rite of farewell" (Grinberg and Grinberg 1989,
p. 157), precludes anticipatory mourning, and complicates subsequent adaptation. The traumatic circumstances responsible for his
exit stir up annihilation anxiety and secondary narcissistic rage. The
amount of aggression thus mobilized can hardly be bound by associative reverie; instead it irradiates backwards, and in the process malicious feelings contaminate the positive memories[37] pertaining to the times before the traumatic event. In Wangh's (1992)
words, "the exile's rage against the land which he was forced to
leave makes him repudiate and repress much of the attachments
of the past" (p. 17). The suspicious and half-hearted reception in

---

37. An alternate hypothesis about the absence of nostalgia in exiles is suggested by Ruth Lax. According to her, "nostalgia can only be for something one
loved and where one *was* loved" (Personal communication, January 1999), and
this was not the case with Jews in Poland, for instance. One way to accommodate my views regarding *poisoning of nostalgia* with Lax's view of a true *lack of
nostalgia* is to be found in Volkan's (1999) division of such experiences into three
categories: *lack of nostalgia*, *poisoned nostalgia*, and *healthy nostalgia*.

the host country makes the exile's assimilation arduous. The inability or the unwillingness to revisit one's homeland blocks access to emotional refueling. The child within is orphaned and must reclaim inch by inch the psychic territory lost. This is achieved with the aid of new transferences, introspection, and creativity, as well as old photographs, music, books, relics, and so on. Under such circumstances physical possessions acquire the status of "linking objects" (Volkan 1981) in a mourning process that might last a lifetime and still remain incomplete (Pollock 1989).[38]

Not surprisingly, indulging in nostalgic ruminations seems a psychic luxury to the exile. The place left is so hated that one neither wishes to nor perhaps can idealize it, even retrospectively. The inner object world is thus split and, in an act of ironic retribution, the earlier positive representations of the land are themselves sent into an intrapsychic exile. The sweet element of the bittersweet pleasure of nostalgia is lost, leaving nothing but bitterness. Yet another factor that precludes the exile from feeling nostalgia is his guilt. Like the immigrant, he feels guilty over success and affluence—but unlike the immigrant, he has the additional burden of the "survivor's guilt" (Niederland 1968). After all, many of his kin have perished under the circumstances that he has fled. This more powerful core of guilt prevents him from enjoying nostalgic regression. There is an adaptive reason for not feeling nostalgia, too. "The impossibility of returning concentrates all one's efforts in the direction of integration with the new surroundings" (Grinberg and Grinberg 1989, p. 147). Together, these traumatic, guilty, and adaptive reasons deprive the exile of the capacity to retrospectively idealize his homeland and use this exalted view as a handy defense against frustrations in his current life. I call this phenomenon "the poisoning of nostalgia." Mali Mann (personal communication, January 1999) provides the following poignant illustration of such a situation:

---

38. The availability of a proxy base for emotional and spiritual refueling (e.g., the state of Israel for East European Jewish migrants to, say, the United States, might prevent such frozen grief.

An uncle of mine left Iran in exile around the time of the Revolution. He has not been able to connect with his good memories of pre-Revolutionary times. Furthermore, he showed hypercathexis over the death of one of our relatives in Iran; he grieved for a much longer period of time than would be expected, and with an exaggerated intensity. Also, the way in which he chose to flee was traumatic in that he had to renounce his last name and take on a new one. In fact, he was forced to adopt this new name for a period of time before leaving his country with false identification. Upon arrival in Paris (where he lived for three years en route to the U.S.), he recaptured his own real name and identity. It is interesting to speculate about what adaptive mechanisms he might have employed in adjusting to a new country, and how he might have compared that lifestyle with the one he had left in his homeland. To this day, after sixteen years of life in the U.S., my uncle has trouble talking about the past and his good memories of the pre-Revolutionary era. At times in conversation, he displays angry feelings and a sense of rejection. The idealization of the past, which I have observed in some immigrant patients in psychotherapy or psychoanalysis, does not seem to exist in his particular case.

At other times, however, the picture is more mixed, nostalgia coexisting with poisoning of nostalgia. Brenner (1999) describes such an occurrence in a middle-aged survivor of the Holocaust who

was eager to forget about his past and make a new life. He married an American woman, started a family and took whatever work he could get. Several years later, he bought his first house, and was completely oblivious until his archival interviews that the neighboring chemical industrial complex visible from his front door was chillingly reminiscent of the I. G. Farber complex back in the concentration camp. Trying to get as far as possible from conscious reminders of the Holocaust, he did not surround himself with other immigrants, refugees, or fellow survivors. However, his periodic reunions with his two friends were enormously important to him. . . . Much to the confusion of his children, he would delight in taking them to German restaurants and German-style festivals where, conversing in German, he tried to regain some version of the good times from long ago. His eyes would light up recalling the tasty

delicacies from his childhood, a time when he freely played games
with his friends and looked forward to a good life. [p. 150]

In contrast, the ordinary immigrant clings to the fantasy of a lost
paradise. Such fantasy expresses a position whereby primary objects are neither given up through the work of grieving nor assimilated into the ego through identification. The result is a temporal
fracture of the psyche. This can, at times, manifest in the
immigrant's fervent plans to "someday" (Akhtar 1991, 1994) return to his homeland; fantasies of retirement and even burial in
one's country of origin are temporally further displaced versions
of this wish. With such a dynamic shift, the future comes to be idealized, robbing the present, once again, of full commitment. Often the "if only" and "someday" fantasies coexist, with nostalgia
providing the fuel for the hope of return.[39]

The temporal direction of the "if only" and "someday" fantasies
differs but their message is essentially the same. Also, while their
conscious focus is upon immigration, both fantasies clearly contain ontogenetically earlier issues. At its bottom, the "if only" fantasy says: "I wish the day had not come when I lost the blissful symbiotic dual unity with my mother nor the day when I became aware
of sexual differences and oedipal boundaries." The "someday"
fantasy says: "A day will come when I will recapture the lost mother
of symbiosis and overcome the sexual and oedipal barriers." The
former attitude fixates the immigrant in the past, the latter in the
future. Both cause a temporal discontinuity in the self experience
(Akhtar 1984, 1992b). The revered Chilean poet Gabriela Mistral
(1889–1957) has captured the essence of such psychic fracture in
the following lines of her poem "The Immigrant Jew."

---

39. In discussing Freud's love of England, Ivan Ward (1993), the educational
director of the Freud Museum in London, touches upon many factors, one of
which echoes the "if only" or "someday" connection mentioned here. Ward states,
"It appears, then, that Freiberg was an encapsulated ideal in the past, and that
England was an ideal 'other place' in the future. . . . Freud's journey to England,
therefore, may also have been a return to something; a return to some idyllic
fantasy of childhood" (p. 38).

I am two. One looks back,
the other turns to the sea.
The nape of my neck seethes with good-byes
and my breast with yearning. [p. 49]

A similar sentiment is encountered in the following lines of "Memories," by Rodrigo Diaz-Perez (1986), who has immigrated to the United States from Paraguay:

And when I arrived he said:
"Don't say, brother,
that you departed.
You will not depart, brother
Though you may leave." [p. 126]

With progressive de-idealization of lost objects, however, meaningful living in the present becomes possible. This does not imply a total renunciation of past objects, only of their hypercathexis. Indeed, continued updating of and ongoing psychic dialogue with the past (Erikson 1950a, Lichtenstein 1963) are not only inevitable but necessary for healthy psychic functioning. However, in such instances, past and future do not replace today; they enrich it.

FROM YOURS OR MINE TO OURS

The Japanese person would feel uncomfortable in thinking of his "self" as something separable from his role. To actualize oneself is to fulfill one's family and social group expectations. In a traditionally oriented Japanese mind, to be "individualistic" in a Western moral sense would almost be equal to being "selfish" in the worst sense of the term. Japanese tend to equate "individualism" (kojinshugi) with "selfishness" (rkoshugi). [Yamamoto and Wagatsuma 1980, p. 123]

Shortly after my landing in the United States I received a rejection to an application for an internship from a southern hospital worded as follows: "We have

> found that persons not of our denomination do not
> feel comfortable working here." A similar letter was
> sent to my wife and me from an Adirondack moun-
> tain resort. Still later, when we purchased a vacation
> home in Connecticut, we were quickly informed that
> the nearby country club (to which we had no inten-
> tions of applying) would not admit Jews. [Wangh
> 1992, p. 16]

In an extension of Mahler's observations regarding the symbiotic dual unity gradually yielding to self- and object differentiation, Bergman (1980) suggests that the sense of "mine" and
"yours" develops out of an earlier sense of "ours." She adds that
the feeling of "we" is "psychically experienced as the 'me' of primary narcissism which still dominates the symbiosis. Only gradually does this archaic 'we' experience develop to include differentiated 'me' and 'we' experience" (p. 205). While I understand
this formulation, my notions about the development of mutuality follow an opposite trajectory. Or perhaps I am simply referring to Bergman's "differentiated 'we'" experience. True mutuality, codified through "we" and "ours," while containing symbiotic
roots, has additional developmental origins. Klein's (1937) views
about the child's dawning sense of gratitude toward the mother,
and Winnicott's (1963) notions about the development of the
capacity for concern are pertinent in this regard. The experience
of sharing the parents (and even aspects of one's own personality characteristics) with siblings also contributes to the capacity
for mutuality (Akhtar and Kramer 1999). More importantly, a
successful resolution of the oedipal phase consolidates the capacity for mutuality ("my mother is also your wife," or "my father is
also your husband"; "we share him/her"). This sketchy ontogen-
esis of mutuality demonstrates that the real "we" follows "mine"
and "yours" and lays the groundwork for elucidating the immigrant's struggles in this area.

For a considerable time after his arrival in the new land, the
immigrant resorts to a "mine" and "yours" split. It is only by resolv-
ing this split that he can experience "ours." Until then, customs,
food, language, games, and moral values are seen as either "mine"

or "yours." An important vehicle in the move toward "we-ness" and the associated identity change is the filling in of the "transitional area" (Winnicott 1953) by local culture. The immigrant's starting to enjoy the movies, literature, and games of his new country heralds such a move. They provide him a ready-made zone of mutual interest with the "foreigners" of his new country. A second medium that facilitates cultural mutuality is the progressive alteration of the immigrant's superego in an encounter with externally changed prohibitions and sanctions. The situation is akin to adolescence (Blos 1967, Erikson 1950b), though clearly the drive upsurge is only relative and mobilized by altered realities. An instinctually more permissive society might at first cause anxiety in the immigrant owing to the threat to his ego stability. Then a liquid phase might set in, during which experimentations with new id freedoms fluctuate with retributions from the "imported" superego. Gradually, these dynamic shifts give way to structural alteration with the deployment of new ego defenses, softening of the superego, and a change in its "cultural character" (Blum 1985, p. 893). The immigrant's notions about right and wrong shift and come to be in greater accordance with the culture at large.[40] The finding of Hojat and colleagues (1999) that Iranians in the United States hold more permissive attitudes toward premarital sex, sexual education, and homosexuality than Iranians in Iran is an example of this type of superego modification. Such structural change enhances the immigrant's capacity for empathy with the residents of his adoptive country. This, in turn, facilitates the development of mutuality and deeper social affiliation.[41]

---

40. In an application of the Russian thinker Mikhail Bakhtin's (1986, 1990) theory of "dialogism" to cross-cultural hermeneutics, Harris (1993) notes that the encounter between the immigrant and his adopted culture is not one-sided. The impact upon the immigrant is clearer. However, the culture itself is affected and inherently altered by the newcomer's interpretation of it.

41. Using a multidimensional approach (psychodynamic, behavioral, body-oriented, creative arts, and cognitive) to treatment, Santini (1999) has illustrated the gradual development of mutuality and empathy-for-the-other in a deeply traumatized refugee.

The most important vehicle for emergence of "we-ness" is, however, the acquisition of (or increased idiomatic fluency in) a new language. In light of this, the paucity of psychoanalytic literature on polylingualism and polyglottism is striking. This is even more remarkable since (1) large numbers of early analysts were analyzed in languages other than their mother tongue, (2) most analysts read Freud's writings in their translated version, (3) many of us have experience with being analyzed in or conducting analysis in a language that is not our mother tongue, or with analyzing patients whose mother tongue is other than ours, and (4) most importantly, words form such an important medium of communication in our enterprise. The early contributions of Ferenczi (1911) and Stengel (1939), the later work of Buxbaum (1949) and Greenson (1950 1954), the more recent essay by Flegenheimer (1989), and a most outstanding monograph by Amati-Mehler and colleagues (1993) on this topic are exceptions in this regard.

The journey from speaking only one's mother tongue, through an introject-like (Kernberg 1976) use of a new language, to true bilingualism is as difficult as it is salutary. Early in this journey, the native language can become an object of idealization with the narcissistic illusion that only it can express things well (Grinberg and Grinberg 1989, Stengel 1939). Its "sonorous wrapping" (Anzieu 1976) is tenaciously clung to; after all the mother tongue is a link to the earliest maternal imago. The new language is devalued as being weak and ridiculous. Consequently, the immigrant lives in two linguistic worlds, pronouncing his own name in two different ways, and switching with relief to his mother tongue after the workday is over. However, the pain of such polyglottism[42] adds to the splitting of self-representations. François Cheng (1985), a Chinese émigré to France who did not know a word of French

---

42. Amati-Mahler and colleagues (1993) distinguish polylingualism from polyglottism. The former refers to the acquisition of various languages, often simultaneously, throughout childhood. The latter refers to learning of a new language later in life, based predominantly on translation, and with much less emotional connotation than the early natural acquisition of a language.

until age 20, eloquently describes such a linguistic cleavage of his self.[43] The same pain is reflected by Julia Kristeva (1988):

> Not to speak your own mother tongue. To live with sounds, logics, that are separated from the nocturnal memory of the body, from the sweet-sour sleep of childhood. To carry within yourself like a secret crypt or like a handicapped child—loved and useless—that language of once-upon-a-time that fades and won't make up its mind to leave you ever. You learn to use another instrument, like express-ing yourself in algebra or on the violin. You can become a virtuoso in this new artifice that provides you with a new body, just as false, sublimated—some would say sublime. You have the impression that the new language is your resurrection: a new skin, a new sex. But the illusion is torn apart when you listen to yourself—on a recorded tape, for example—and the melody of your own voice comes back to you in a bizarre way, from nowhere, closer to the grumble of the past than to the [linguistic] code of today. . . . Thus, between two languages, your element is silence. [p. 20; in Amati-Mehler et al. 1993, pp. 264–265]

The theme of an inner linguistic slaughter also finds its way in the following lines of "Conversations with God About My Present Whereabouts," a poem by Reinzi Crusz (1995), a Sri-Lankan im-migrant to Canada:

> The chameleon
> has muted my rowdy scream
> to the whisper of a white-boned land,
> and stretching in silence,
> I am a king of silence. [p. 44]

---

43. In a less dramatic vein, Freud also expressed a similar emotion. Soon after his arrival in England, he wrote to Raymond de Saussere, the Swiss psychoana-lyst who had congratulated him on his escape: "Perhaps, you have omitted the one point that the emigrant feels so particularly painfully. It is—one can only say—the loss of the language in which one had lived and thought, and which one will never be able to replace with another for all one's efforts at empathy" (Freud, June 11, 1938, quoted in Gay [1988], p. 632).

A more optimistic note, however, is struck by the writer Eva Hoffman (1989), who describes her inner translations from her native Polish to English, which she had to learn because of immigration.

> [In] my translation therapy, I keep [going] back and forth over the rifts, not to heal them but to see that [I]—one person, first person singular—have been on both sides. Patiently, I use English as a conduit to go back and down, all the way down to childhood, almost to the beginning. When I learn to say those smallest, first things in the language that has served for detachment and irony and abstraction, I begin to see where the languages I've spoken have their correspondences—how I can move between them without being split by the difference. [p. 273]

Perhaps the degree to which a linguistically lacerated self can be healed is variable.[44] However, mending is in evidence with an increasing dominance of the acquired language, which begins to appear in spontaneous humor, dreams and in talking during sleep. Another indicator of linguistic identity change is when the immigrant begins to treat obscenities and the terms for genitals and curses in his new language with an instinctual and moral valence comparable to that invested in similar words of his mother tongue. For a long time, the immigrant's unblinking use of obscenities in his acquired language neither provides him a gratifying id discharge nor causes him a noticeable superego admonishment. ("When you say 'fuck' it doesn't sound dirty, but when I say 'fuck'

---

44. Eugène Ionesco, Vladimir Nabokov, Samuel Beckett, and Salman Rushdie are four immigrant writers who show four completely different attitudes in this regard. Ionesco never wrote in his mother tongue and chose French instead to express his creativity. Nabokov moved in succession from a mastery of Russian, French, and German to English, in which he wrote his best-known works. Beckett "migrated" to French and after many years returned to writing in his native English (see Casement [1982] for Beckett's relationship with his mother tongue). Rushdie freely sprinkles his English text with Urdu/Hindi colloquialisms from India and thus creates a hybrid language of his own.

it sounds dirty," said a perceptive medical student to me some fifteen years ago!) For "real" cursing, the immigrant uses his native language only. Gradually, however, as the associative networks of both languages begin to interdigitate, the later-acquired obscenities too gather affective valence, though perhaps never truly equal in degree to that of obscene words in the mother tongue (Ferenczi 1911).

Two more things need to be considered: (1) that different self-representations might still continue to be under the influence of different languages and express different conflicts (developmentally earlier and later?), ego skills (e.g., mathematics), and aspirations,[45] and (2), that adopting a second language might at times represent the acquisition of a developed identity for the first time. Amati-Mehler and colleagues (1993), who have authored the most searching psychoanalytic investigation of languages so far, conclude that

> a multilingual dimension certainly does allow for an internal enrichment [and] not only at the cognitive level. However, it is also true that the actual mental organization of the multilingual subject lends itself in particular to the enacting of defenses, splittings, and repressions. Occasionally a new language represents a lifesaving anchor which allows for "rebirth." At other times it can be a justification for the mutilation of the internal world of the self. [p. 108]

Interestingly, in most writings on the issue of language, it is speaking as against being spoken to that is emphasized. The fact, however, is that constantly being talked to in a language other than one's mother tongue is also burdensome. No one has captured this sort of agony better than the New York–based Urdu poet, Sudhir Chopra.

---

45. Could this partly explain the fact that unlike great prose, great poetry, which draws heavily on the prosodic qualities of a language, has never been written in a later-acquired language?

Mujh se zaban-e-ghair mein jo guftgu karey
Kya khaak zakhm-e-dil ko mere rafu karey[46]

[The one who talks to me in a language other than
that of my heart
How, tell me, can he heal the splits and wounds that
inhabit its dark corners]
(personal communication, 1999)

SOME CAVEATS

If a man will begin with certainties, he shall end in
doubts; but if he will be content to begin with doubts,
he shall end in certainties. [Francis Bacon]

Caveat: (L. *caveat*, let him beware, 3rd pers. sing.
pres. subj. of *cavere*, to behave, take heed): a warning, admonition. [*Webster's New Universal Unabridged
Dictionary*, second edition (1983), p. 289]

Throughout this chapter my emphasis has been on the resolution of the splitting of the self and the object world that tends to
result from immigration. I have proposed that mending of such
splits in four dimensions—drives and affects, space, time, and social affiliation—is what leads to a psychic rebirth, the emergence
of a new and hybrid identity. Now I wish to offer some caveats in
order to "soften" the proposed model and render it more realistic. *First,* the four dynamic progressions described earlier are neither independent of each other nor exhaustive. There might be
dimensions that I have failed to include, even recognize. *Second,*
these developmental tracks do not have clear end-points. The identity change of immigration continues to evolve throughout the life
span. *Third,* the progression outlined here is characteristic only of

---

46. By now, it may be evident that in quoting poetry I have cited originals
for only those poems that were in my mother tongue, Urdu. To be sure, this is
a bit partisan. However, it is also because I had little faith in my translations and
therefore wanted to let the poets speak for themselves.

uncomplicated cases where the capacity for intrapsychic separateness existed before immigration, where there was at least some choice in leaving one's country, and where the host country was more or less welcoming. However, in instances where the pre-immigration character structure is problematic, where migration is forced and the possibility of revisiting the country does not exist, and where a good-enough holding environment is not found in the new land, the mourning necessary for such psychological advance might not be feasible. *Fourth,* it remains unclear whether the identity that does emerge as a result of the mourning–liberation process of immigration is a reasonably solid hybrid entity or a loose albeit well-functioning confederacy of diverse selves. Garza-Guerrero (1974) advances the former view. He states that

> A new identity will reflect the final consolidation into a remodeled ego identity of those selective identifications with the new culture which were harmoniously integrated or fitted in with the past cultural heritage. What actually ensues from the crisis of culture shock, if adequately solved, is a fecund growth of the self. What began as a threat to identity, mourning, and low self-esteem ends in a confirmation of both ego identity and self-esteem. [p. 425]

A less sanguine, postmodernist view is expressed by Copelman (1993) who states that

> Instead of positing unified, discrete cultures and nations to which we can all someday claim to belong, recent works suggest that we are bound to have fragmented allegiances, and dissonant voices within ourselves that name our world. This is not, I believe, some new version of the melting pot, for that assumes a synthesis which seems not only overly idealistic, but in fact undesirable. Instead of synthesis, there is the frightening but also exciting potential of multiplicity. Instead of completion or closure, there is the anxiety of partial identities as well as the challenge of ongoing process. [p. 79]

In my own socioclinical experience, the hybrid identity that emerges as a consequence of advance along these four lines is not a rock-like structure. Indeed, in certain psychosocial realms one or the other self-representation continues to predominate. Searles's (1986) reminder that a healthy identity does not possess a monolithic solidity is pertinent here. Eisnitz's (1980) view of a well-functioning self as made up of subsets of self-representations with variable proximity to affect, action, and fantasy also speaks to this point.

This may be accompanied by a mixed sense of belonging to multiple places while at the same time not truly belonging to any of them. In a poignant description of such inner psychic experience of the immigrant, Anni Bergman states:

> I love my home. I have put a lot into it. But is it really home? Home, as Winnicott says, is where we come from. When I go to Vienna I always go to the house where I was born and lived for twenty years. Is it home? It isn't. So in a certain way I don't have a home, but feel at home in many places. Emigration means among many other things being at home in at least two languages and maybe in many places. Having family and friends in many places, it also means to me, I think, an eternal longing to belong which is never quite fulfilled. I "belong" to several analytic groups. I don't fully belong to any one. Only my children and grandchildren, who certainly don't belong to me, do I really belong to. [personal communication, May 1999]

Finally, it is the intrapsychic meaning that various self- and object representations come to acquire, the resistance purpose (including defensive functions against drive derivatives) served by shifts in them, their adaptive aspects, and their vivid or concealed unfolding in the transference–countertransference axis, that is of technical significance to our work as psychotherapists and analysts (Holmes 1992).

SUMMARY

> A man who sets out to make himself up is taking on the Creator's role, according to one way of seeing things; he's unnatural, a blasphemer, an abomination of abominations. From another angle, you could see pathos in him, heroism in his struggle, in his will-

ingness to risk: not all mutants survive. [Rushdie
1989, p. 49]

This chapter describes the phenomenology and psychodynam-
ics of the identity change consequent upon immigration. It delin-
eates four interlinked strands in such transformation. These tracks
(and their associated metaphoric journeys) involve the dimensions
of drive and affects (from love or hate to ambivalence), interpersonal and psychic space (from near or far to optimal distance),
temporality (from yesterday or tomorrow to today), and social affiliation (from yours or mine to ours). Issues of idealization and
devaluation, closeness and distance, hope and regret, vulnerability to inordinate nostalgia as well as incapacity to experience nostalgia, the transitional areas of the mind, superego modification,
mutuality, and linguistic transformation are addressed.

The related themes of loss, wistfulness, temporal fracture, lexi-
cal cleavage, and cultural anomie are elaborated in my 1982 poem
(written nine years after my arrival in this country) entitled "A
World Without Seasons."

In the greedy flim-flam
For two worlds, we have lost the one in hand.
And now,
Like the fish who chose to live on a tree,
We writhe in foolish agony.
Our Gods reduced to grotesque exhibits.
Our poets, mute, pace in the empty halls of our conversation.
The silk of our mother tongue banned from the fabric
Of our dreams,
And now,
We hum the national anthem but our
Pockets do not jingle with the coins of patriotism.
Barred from weddings and funerals,
We wear good clothes to no avail.
Proudly we mispronounce our own names,
And those of our monuments and our children.
Forsaking the gray abodes and sunken graves of
Our ancestors, we have come to live in
A world without seasons.

The sadness of it all (at least at the time of its writing) notwithstanding, the salutary aspects of the fact that I was able to put my
feelings in a newly acquired idiom must not be overlooked.[47] Such
paradox is also evident in the tension between the view that the
mourning–liberation process of immigration results in a reconsoli-
dated hybrid identity and the view that the result of such a process
is a contextually resilient confederation of self-representations. To
be sure, a clear-cut resolution or balance between these two positions is not possible. It is the intrapsychic meanings of various self-
and object representations and their resistance and adaptive purposes that are of technical significance to our work as therapists.

---

47. Note also the distinction between my two immigration poems. The first,
"Two Homes" (p. 82) was written a few years earlier than the second, "A World
Without Seasons" (p. 105). Not only is the second one characterized by greater
suppleness of language and experiential breadth, the affects of sadness and irony
are more prominent in it as against those of anger and cynicism that pervade
the first poem.

Part III

CROSS-CULTURAL TREATMENT

4

PSYCHOANALYSIS AND PSYCHODYNAMIC PSYCHOTHERAPY

Earlier notions regarding the nonapplicability of psychoanalysis and psychoanalytically derived psychotherapies to non-Western and ethnic minority patients (DeVos 1980, Hsu 1953, Neki 1975, Obendorf 1950, Surya and Jayaram 1964) have recently come under increasing challenge. Arguments previously forwarded that such patients lacked sufficient individuation, did not have the capacity for self-reflectiveness and introspection, subscribed to animistic belief systems, and were enmeshed with their families of origin and their internalized dictates, are now either deemed invalid or regarded as not constituting major contraindications to psychoanalytic treatment. An increasing recognition of the ethnocentric biases of psychoanalytic developmental postulates and treatment methodology (Moskowitz 1996, Pérez Foster 1996, Rendon 1996, Roland 1988, 1996), as well as an emergent theoretical and technical pluralism in psychoanalysis (Akhtar 1999d, Pulver 1993, Strenger 1989, Wallerstein 1990) are together responsible for a greater spirit of clinical experimentation. Renewed vigor is evident, and reports that psychoanalytic psychotherapy and even psychoanalysis proper might be beneficially applicable to Indian (Bonovitz and Ergas 1999, Kakar 1985, Mehta 1998, Roland 1988), Chinese (Ng 1985), Japanese (Doi 1973, Roland 1988), Latin American

(Bonovitz and Ergas 1999, Ticho 1971), Korean (Smolar 1999), and other immigrant populations (Akhtar 1995a) are becoming increasingly available.

However, most of the contributors listed above tend to qualify their assertions by suggesting occasional modifications of technique. Such modifications range from accommodating the ego-syntonic cultural bents of patients to innovative analytic interventions that deal with intrapsychic conflicts specific to these patient groups. I myself (Akhtar 1995a) have delineated various technical guidelines for conducting in-depth psychotherapeutic work or psychoanalysis with immigrants.

In this chapter, I synthesize the scattered literature and extend my earlier views in this regard. I present eight guidelines for working with immigrant patients and illustrate them with the help of clinical vignettes. These are only guidelines, however; they are not to replace the customary work of transference interpretation, reconstruction, and countertransference vigilance. Nor are these suggestions meant to interfere with the "trio of guideposts" (Pine 1997, p. 13) of abstinence, neutrality, and anonymity that are a cornerstone of our work. What follows are neither rigid rules nor necessary in all cases. Indeed, the more psychologically sophisticated and "analyzable" the patient, the less attention need be paid to these guidelines. In less sophisticated patients and in treatments leaning more toward psychotherapy, these guidelines warrant greater attention. It might not be out of place to add that, for me, psychoanalysis and psychoanalytic psychotherapy are closely blended. My credo in this regard is akin to that of Pine (1997), who states

> I often think of my clinical work in terms of doing as much psycho-analysis as possible in context where I do as much psychotherapy as necessary—the latter being precisely what makes it possible to pursue the former. At other times, or with other patients, the psycho-therapeutic portions seem a full partner of equal status and value in the enterprise. I do not quite think of these latter treatments as psychoanalysis, but I cannot think of them as *not* psychoanalysis, since psychoanalysis inevitably enters into the work so significantly for an analyst. [p. 3, original italics]

In either case, however, these guidelines do constitute an important background[48] for the "evenly suspended attention" (Freud 1912, p. 111) mandatory for our work. It is with such caveats that we may now consider the following technical guidelines for treating immigrant patients in intensive psychotherapy or psychoanalysis.

TECHNICAL GUIDELINES

> External social factors such as prejudice, racism, sexism, poverty, and social disadvantage—all of which cause profound pain, perhaps most especially for Black and ethnic minority patients because of the situations they find themselves in—are real and must be taken into account as vital clinical concerns. [Kareem 1992, p. 20]

> Arab patients in Israel have only recently begun to seek modern forms of outpatient psychotherapy. . . . in light of the political antagonism between Jews and Arabs, it is understandable that at times, both therapist and patient may attempt to avoid discussion of their cultural differences. [Gorkin 1996, pp. 161, 163]

Maintaining Cultural Neutrality and Avoiding Countertransference Pitfalls

Among the guidelines for working with culturally diverse immigrant patients, maintaining cultural neutrality and avoiding countertransference pitfalls easily rank at the top. *Cultural neutrality* refers to the analyst's capacity to remain equidistant from the values, ideals, and mores of the patient's culture and those of his own. This sounds like a tall order and yet there is no escaping the fact

---

48. "A background," said the eminent British photographer Lord Snowdon, "has to be just this side of being something, and just the other side of being nothing" (Lacayo 1984, p. 54).

that the analyst must strive to achieve such an ego position. Being human and belonging to a particular racial, cultural, and political group, the analyst undeniably has a certain ethnic dimension to his identity and this is indeed normal (see Chapter 2). Such ethnic components of identity develop from both the internalization of family and group legacies ("we do this") *and* the repudiation of unacceptable instinctual residues ("we don't do this, they do"). The more aggressively charged these residues are and the greater the narcissistic injuries inflicted by ongoing external realities, the more forceful and hate-ridden the projections of one's inner "badness" become. This essentially is the basis of prejudice, a regressive pathway the analyst must avoid at all costs. However, the analyst cannot and must not attempt to erase the ethnic component of his own identity. Perhaps it might be useful to illustrate all this with a simple example. Matters are fine if an analyst feels greater affinity with a particular variety of his patient's headdress (e.g., a Sikh's *pagdi*, a Jew's *yarmulke*, an Arab's *kaffiyeh*) but there is a problem at hand if the analyst regards the others as inherently bizarre. Cultural neutrality can coexist with ethnicity, not with discrimination.

The development and maintenance of genuine cultural neutrality can be facilitated by the following five measures. *First* and foremost, the analyst's own analysis would, one hopes, reduce the internal aggression to the extent that major projective defenses would no longer be essential for his character organization. However, since most training analyses (and intensive psychotherapies of psychotherapists) in this country are conducted in homoethnic dyads, it is possible that certain areas of ethnic, racial, and religious prejudice might remain unexamined in such treatment. Treatment might end with such prejudices sequestered but quite intact. The onus then comes to be upon the therapist himself, especially once he begins treating culturally diverse patients.

Second, didactic courses on culture should be included in psychoanalytic and psychotherapeutic curricula. Such courses should seek to highlight the myriad ways in which cultural, racial, and ethnic differences give shape and content to the transference–countertransference events (Abbasi 1997, Akhtar 1995a, 1998b, Fischer 1971, Goldberg et al. 1974, Holmes 1992, 1994, Mehta

1998, Ticho 1971, Zaphiropoulos 1982). Such courses might include didactic sessions as well as experiential workshops. Admittedly, one is training therapists and analysts, not social anthropologists, but it remains important that the trainees acquire sensitivity to a variety of psychosocial facets of cultural diversity. Kraft-Goin (1999) illustrates this with convincing clinical examples and Taylor (1989) offers a formidable list of what one needs to know in this regard:

> Family structure. Important events in the life cycle. Roles of individual members. Rules of interpersonal interactions. Communication and linguistic rules. Rules of decorum and discipline. Religious beliefs. Standards for health and hygiene. Food preferences. Dress and personal appearance. History and traditions. Holidays and celebrations. Education and teaching methods. Perceptions of work and play. Perceptions of time and space. Explanations of natural phenomena. Attitudes towards pets and animals. Artistic and musical values and tastes. Life expectations and aspirations. [pp. 18–19]

Such courses, especially if given while the trainee is still in his own treatment, can mobilize a scrutiny of one's biases and prejudices, often with salutary results. It is therefore encouraging to see that psychotherapy and psychoanalytic training programs are now beginning to include courses on cross-cultural sensitivity.

A *third* way to cultivate the cultural neutrality is for the analyst to open himself to the "intercultural challenge" (Kareem 1992, p. 30) of taking on as many patients from diverse cultures as possible. Overcoming the initial all-too-human resistance of xenophobia can only enrich the analyst's inner world of feelings and knowledge. Such experience would also sensitize him to the cultural nuances in personality structure and functioning as well as to the fundamental universality that exists beneath human diversity.

Fourth, cultural neutrality also requires that the analyst avoid excessive curiosity about the patient's culture. Gorkin (1996) notes that in the treatment of culturally diverse patients

> One of the typical areas of countertransference difficulty is the therapist's pervasive, and occasionally hovering, curiosity about the

patient's cultural background. The therapist seizes upon the opportunity to meet a representative of [an] intriguing foreign culture,
and in the process loses sight of the therapeutic task. Cultural material is explored more for its intrinsic interest than for its immediate relevance to the patient. [pp. 161–162]

Finally, those therapists and analysts who live in cosmopolitan
areas and maintain ongoing social dialogue, if not personal friendships, with people of diverse cultures generally may be better able
to maintain cultural neutrality in their clinical work. Experience
increases knowledge and facilitates empathy.

In essence the therapist's (1) personal treatment to mitigate
paranoid defenses, (2) study of the interface of social anthropology with clinical work, (3) treating patients of many cultures, (4)
avoiding the pitfall of excessive culturalization of the analytic ego,
and (5) leading an open, cosmopolitan life, will together help
develop and maintain cultural neutrality. Compromise of this capacity, especially when marked and directed at those seeking help
for their mental suffering is "antihumanity and in the widest sense
anti-sanity" (Kareem 1992, p. 21).

Judiciously Accommodating the Therapeutic Framework
to Cultural Differences

Psychoanalytic and psychotherapeutic sessions are time-limited.
They begin and end at set times. Such firm boundaries are implicit
assertions of the reality principle (Freud 1911) and guardians of
separateness, and of the incest barrier at a deeper, unconscious
level. It is against the backdrop of such limits that the patient's
needs, wishes, and demands for transcendence and transgression
unfold and are understood, renounced, modified, and rechan-
neled. Punctuality for sessions is not merely ritualistic window dressing. It has deep meanings.

At the same time, it can hardly be denied that the experience of
time is governed by forces of the culture at large. Hence, it might
not be easily transportable across national and cultural boundaries.
Pande (1968) has eloquently summarized the difference between

East and West in the time experience; the same, by and large, applies to most less industrialized, third-world countries.

> For the East, relatively speaking, past, present, and future merge
> into one another; for the West they are discrete entities. For the
> East, experience in time is like water collected in a pool (stagnant
> perhaps); for the West, time is more like water flowing in a stream,
> and one is acutely aware that what flows away, flows away forever.
> [pp. 428–429]

Holding a time perspective that is fundamentally different from
that of his country of adoption, the East-to-West immigrant might
appear temporally slovenly while the West-to-East immigrant might
appear unduly concerned about schedules. As might be suspected,
this difference has deep roots. In industrialized nations, time was
gradually rendered into a commodity. Passing moments were captured, named, measured, and sold. Like water, time was put into a
tray and frozen into ice cubes of designated length. Each cube had
its price, depending upon the size. Hiring of labor, operation of
production lines, rental of property, all became time-dependent
and tied to capital generation. Efficiency and punctuality became
nearly synonymous. Thus was born what I call the *time of the mind*
or the *time of money*. In contrast, the nonindustrialized nations,
where planes, trains, phones, faxes, and e-mail did not create rapid
access to others and where the manufacture of commodities did
not take over the community, the beginning and ending of various social get-togethers continued to depend upon the arrival of
loved ones (often by treacherously unreliable means) and the
permissive winks of gods and seasons. Action began only when the
libido–aggression balance in the social matrix shifted in favor of
the former. This is what I call the *time of the heart* or the *time of love*.
    When someone from a third-world country migrates to an in-
dustrialized country, he carries within himself the *time of the heart*
but has to adapt to the *time of the mind*. What therefore appears as
a lack of punctuality in such circumstances might still be punctuality but to a different internal clock. Similarly, when someone from
an industrialized nation immigrates to a third-world country, he

carries within himself the *time of the mind* but has to adapt to the *time of the heart*. What then appears an inordinate and rigid reliance on punctuality is merely a matter of loyalty to a different inner sense of time. There is in the end, it seems, a *bicultural punctuality* that needs to be empathized with while dealing with all immigrant individuals.

The analyst must therefore keep in mind that there may exist discrepancies in the experience of time and in the conventions used to manage time between his and the patient's society of origin. What constitutes punctuality varies cross-culturally and even within subcultures (Antokoletz 1993, Lager and Zwerling 1980). Such awareness will enhance the analyst's empathic ability to distinguish between a culturally determined trivial lateness for sessions from a meaningful "attack on the analytic process" (Limentani 1989, p. 252).[49]

Similar considerations might apply to the degree of deference the patient might show toward his or her therapist. Recognizing distinctions of degrees in this realm might help the therapist explore, rather than take on face value, an immigrant patient's quick agreement to pay the stated fee, for instance. It can enhance empathy with those immigrant patients who, even in their intrapsychic life, never refer to their analysts by first names. It can also lead to "necessary technical alterations" (Pine 1998, p. 73) or, at least, to some changes in the formalities surrounding the treatment.

Case 1

After his North American analyst would say "Come on in," a recently migrated Japanese young man would walk up to the office door and stop there, hesitating. The analyst would then say "Come on in" again, and only then would the patient truly walk into the office. Finding it a bit puzzling, and even annoying, the

---

49. For an unusual and thought-provoking discussion of making exceptions to the temporal framework of psychoanalytic sessions, see Kurtz (1988).

analyst decided to learn more about Japanese culture and, in the process, gathered that his patient was behaving in accordance with his native culture. There was nothing odd in his feeling the need to be invited twice, first from the waiting room to the door and then into the office. The analyst decided to train himself to behave accordingly rather than force his patient into a false and inauthentic compliance.

The analyst's resilience in this case certainly seems exemplary. Less dramatic examples are perhaps more common. These might include a North American analyst's beginning to shake hands with his patients at the start and the end of each session after his move to certain parts of Europe and Latin America where this is customary. On the other hand, an analyst who has migrated from those regions to the United States would soon give up the practice in an accommodation to his patients' cultural expectations. At bottom, all this parallels the attitude of devoted parents who accommodate themselves to their offsprings' interests and talents, even though these might differ from their own. This brings up the issue of the parallels that exist between clinical psychoanalysis and psychotherapy on the one hand and good parenting on the other.

Adopting a Developmental Stance
and Conducting Developmental Work

The analyst of an immigrant patient must bear in mind the relatively greater role he plays as a new object. The similarities between the developmental process and the analytic process (Blum 1971, Burland 1986, Escoll 1977, Fleming 1972, Greenacre 1975, Loewald 1960, Schlessinger and Robbins 1983, Settlage 1992, 1993) may be more marked in such analyses. But what is actually meant by a "developmental stance" (Settlage 1992) and "developmental work" (Pine 1997)? The former is fundamentally a generative attitude. It is epitomized by the following extension of Freud's metaphor of the analyst as a sculptor by Loewald (1960): "We bring out the true form by taking away the neurotic distortions. However, as in sculpture, we must have, if only in rudiments, an image of that which needs to be brought into its own" (p. 8).

In other words, besides helping the patient resolve his psychopathology, the analyst also seeks to release the patient's developmental potential. He does so "by establishing a developmental relationship, by expecting development, by encouraging the patient's developmental initiatives, and by acknowledging developmental achievements" (Settlage 1994, p. 42).

Operationalizing this perspective and drawing upon the recent work of Fonagy and Target (1997), Pine (1997) has outlined the following eight constituents of "developmental work": (1) naming of affects, (2) helping the patient find words for inner experiences, (3) confirming the patient's reality, (4) continuing to work with the patient matter-of-factly even in the face of what seems reprehensible to the patient, (5) surviving the patient's assaults, (6) maintaining hope over long periods of time when the patient might feel no reason to remain optimistic, (7) genuinely regarding psychic development to be lifelong, and (8) recognizing that analytic process, "like good parenting" (p. 201), includes both a context of safety and an expectation of autonomous functioning. In this context, it should be remembered that

> with each undoing of some aspect of pathology, there is the opportunity for development in that same area. With each increment of development, the personality structure is strengthened. The strengthened structure increases the patient's tolerance for the therapeutic exposure of repressed, anxiety-creating urges, fantasies, and feelings. Further therapeutic work is followed in turn by more development, and so on. [Settlage 1992, p. 355]

Under ideal circumstances, advances in ego development gradually follow interpretive resolution of conflict. This certainly is more true when the treatment is psychoanalysis. In psychotherapy (and, at times, even in psychoanalysis) of recent immigrants, however, a judicious use of relatively didactic interventions can actually facilitate both ego growth and the patient's capacity for deeper self-examination.

Case 2

A long-haired, gaunt, second-year psychiatry resident who had arrived in the United States from South Korea only fifteen months earlier entered psychoanalysis with an American-born, white, Jewish analyst. His complaints centered around awkwardness in social situations. He felt inhibited in a number of realms. One situation that was especially difficult for him involved placing his order when he and his American classmates went for lunch at restaurants or delis near the hospital. They seemed to know exactly what to order while he became tongue-tied. He did not know how to order things, what certain things were, what food items went together, and so on. As a result, he would lie and try to avoid going for lunch but then he was left hungry. Also, his colleagues were fond of him (since he was outstanding in studies and always forthcoming whenever they needed clinical coverage) and often dragged him along with them.

In his analysis, the anxiety about eating was found to have deeper roots. When he was 6 years old, his mother had died of scleroderma, having become quite emaciated and restricted due to contractures. He had memories of taking home-cooked food to his mother, as she was spending her last days in a village hospital in South Korea. She would often give him portions of food from her plate. Eating and asking for food were thus matters highly charged with early emotional conflicts for him. In the transference, too, he showed little entitlement, little desire to receive love or attention from the analyst. Instead, he felt compelled to be on time, pay promptly, and produce profuse associations (food!) for the analyst who he believed was depressed (sclerodermatic!). As interpretive work proceeded, the patient's inhibition began to relax but the fear of ordering food in restaurants remained. Shame over not knowing what to order was intense and pervasive in his associations.

During one such session, the analyst decided to put aside his usual maneuvers of reconstruction ("How can you allow yourself to eat if the good food is for your mother?") and transference interpretation ("Perhaps you want me to permit you to eat well?"; or, "What about your wishes to take from me? Eat me up?," etc.). Instead, he said "Look, this is the United States. It is a country of immigrants. Lots of people go to restaurants and don't know what this or that particular dish contains. So they ask. They simply ask the waiter: "Excuse me, what exactly is such and such?" Sometimes, they even ask to be shown the particular food! The same applies to you. Nobody will care if you ask. In fact, it is their job to tell you what this or that food is." The patient responded by a profound sense of relief and gratitude. Even though it took him a few efforts to put this fully in practice, he reported feeling immensely helped by this intervention.

Was this an unneeded supportive measure? A manipulative attempt at superego alteration? Clearly, it is possible to view this intervention in such a light. It would then seem that the analyst was saying to the patient: "Go ahead, eat. I give you permission. Your mother would not die because of your eating properly." Viewed in this fashion, the intervention would appear to be a major countertransference enactment. On the other hand, the fact that the patient did not feel inhibited in ordering food when he went to a Korean restaurant in a nearby large city prompts a more sympathetic view of the intervention. Viewed in this alternate manner, the intervention seems to be the provision of an auxiliary ego function[50] rather than a transference manipulation. The latter view is supported by the fact that the essential work of analysis subsequently remained focused upon intrapsychic conflicts and their unfolding in the transference–countertransference axis.

Unmasking and Interpreting the Cultural Rationalizations of Intrapsychic Conflicts and Transference Reactions

Another important task in the treatment of culturally diverse patients involves helping them to disengage cultural differences

---

50. Settlage (1994) suggests that the provision of an "auxiliary regulation pending improvement in the patient's self-regulatory capacity" (p. 48) is highly useful in situations where ego functions are compromised.

from intrapsychic conflicts. Indeed, the two frequently overlap. Intrapsychic issues can make cultural differences appear more problematic. The latter, in turn, can ignite trigger points in the patient's field of emotional vulnerability. Given such dialectical relationship between culture and neurosis, it is not surprising that patients often seek to distance themselves, from the psychic depths as well as from their emerging wishes in the transference, by invoking cultural issues (Abbasi 1997, Akhtar 1995a, Leary 1997). While in this context any uncovering has to be guided by tact (Poland 1975) and by regard for optimal distance (Akhtar 1992a, Bouvet 1958, Escoll 1992), such use of "reality" as a defense must be vigilantly looked for and ultimately handled in an interpretive fashion.

Two clinical examples should highlight the defensive use of culture and its technical handling. In the first instance, the patient's selective deployment of a cultural rationalization turned out to be repudiation of inner psychic life and of her active ownership of it.

Case 3

A married Iranian law student "accidentally" became pregnant soon after converting her psychotherapy into analysis. She reported feeling extremely upset. Though she was certain of not wanting to have a child at this time, she felt that she could not have an abortion. When I asked her what made her hesitate, she retorted that I should know that abortion is prohibited in Islam. Now, having known her for some time, I knew she was hardly an observant Muslim. Indeed, she loved to drink, occasionally smoked cigarettes, and was defiant of other traditional modes of conduct from her culture of origin. As a result, I was surprised by her using a religious explanation for her hesitation to terminate an unwanted pregnancy. Bringing this discrepancy to her attention helped her see that her reluctance to have an abortion was related to a deeper, personal conflict. On the one hand, she wistfully desired to have a child. On the other hand, having just entered law school, she did not want the burden. Exploration of these issues and of the dynamics behind her getting pregnant at this time in the first place, freed her ego to make a relatively remorse-free decision in favor of abortion.

In the second case, rigid externalization of a painful childhood scenario on contemporary cultural realities was used in the service of an intensely sadomasochistic transference.

Case 4

A young Hindu immigrant physician from Bangladesh sought help from a middle-aged Jewish psychoanalyst. He and his wife had just had their first child. The patient was thrilled by this but also found himself suffering from disturbing feelings of envy toward their son, who was receiving "all the love in this world" from his mother. This inwardly shamed him and was a source of great distress for him. The presence of intense maternal hunger and sibling rivalry underneath his Laius-like rage were unmistakable.

The treatment began as psychotherapy and was later converted to psychoanalysis. Symptomatically relieved, the patient began to recount intricate details of his childhood. While very close to his mother, he had suffered an intensely traumatic situation. His older brother, for various reasons, was raised by his aunt but was brought to the paternal home every few months. During the days the older brother stayed there, the patient felt completely forgotten and ignored by his mother and father. They would dote upon the older brother and his own appeals for attention would be met by "But you stay with us all the time and he is here only for a few days." Clearly, this early childhood scenario was casting a heavy shadow on his feelings toward his son.

As the analysis progressed, the patient began to have wishes to enter psychoanalytic training. However, he feared that he would not be accepted for training and, even if accepted, would not be popular and successful in a psychoanalytic institute. Exploration of these fears revealed that he thought that the world of psychoanalysis was dominated by Jews and that non-Jews, like him, were not truly accepted in it. More significantly, the patient felt that his analyst liked his Jewish analysands more than he liked the patient. At first, such concerns were voiced fearfully. However with further analysis of superego resistances, the complaints became vociferous, even mocking and sadomasochistic. The patient began to tease and torture the analyst by repeatedly asking whether the analyst agreed with his idea or not that his not being Jewish stood in the way of his professional success. The analyst's efforts, of course, remained directed at the sadomasochistic transference agenda and its childhood origins in sibling rivalry and the attendant rage toward the parents. The patient occasionally gained insight into this dynamic and the intensity of his litany would diminish. At other times, he would lose this insight and become regressed all over again.

During one such session, the patient again asked the analyst, "Don't you think that I would be more acceptable to the psychoanalytic group if I were Jewish?" Having responded to this question hundreds of times, the analyst decided to say something different: "I think it's possible that you are right." The patient, unexpectedly robbed of his projections, was dumbfounded. After a few moments of silence, the analyst resumed: "Now that I have answered your question on what you believe to be the factual basis, let me ask you a few questions. What satisfaction did you get out of hearing what I said? Also, what connection do you think this satisfaction might have with your wish that your parents confess that they loved your brother more than you? And, finally, since you are so fond of assigning percentages to everything, let me ask you what percentage of what has just transpired, in your opinion, related to your intrapsychic conflicts and what percentage to certain external realities?" It was the last part of the analyst's intervention that gave the patient yet another opportunity to wiggle out of acknowledging that his childhood trauma and resulting sadomasochism were driving his interrogation of the analyst. Neurotically smug all over again, the patient responded: "I think 90 percent of it is reality, and 10 percent neurosis." The analyst firmly countered him by pounding on a nearby table and saying "Wrong! It is 10 percent reality and 90 percent neurosis!"

This vignette demonstrates the vehemence with which intrapsychic conflicts can be externalized and given a seemingly "cultural" cast. However, what is more impressive here is the analyst's technical intervention (even if born out of some countertransference fatigue) of acknowledging a bit of reality in the patient's projection in order to gain access to the patient's intrapsychic conflict. Comparing this case with the one immediately preceding yields an interesting technical guideline. When the tension between the world of external reality and the world of internal perceptions and meanings is "fine and fluctuating" (Abbasi 1997, p. 4), then externalizations can be directly questioned. More intense and tenacious cultural rationalizations, however, require some validation of the kernel of reality in them before becoming amenable to analytic exploration.

Validating Feelings of Dislocation and Facilitating Mourning

The therapist must offer empathic resonance to the immigrant patient's loss of historical continuity and his need for its restoration. The patient's attempts to bridge the gap between his two cultures must find respect and nonjudgmental acceptance in the clinical situation. At times, the therapist might even validate the immigrant's feeling dislocated in the mainstream culture before handling the associative material interpretively or for reconstruction. In cases where the patient has been, or currently is, the recipient of prejudice and discrimination, such "mirroring" (Kohut 1977) and "affirmative" (Killingmo 1989) interventions can have healing effects of their own. Pine's (1997) recent remark that, at times, the seemingly nonspecific elements of technique acquire highly individualized therapeutic effects is pertinent in this context. At the same time, such emphasis on validation, empathy, and affirmation should not make one overlook the fact that for true mourning to occur a lament of loss and dislocation is not enough. True mourning can only occur with the acknowledgment and assimilation of one's own aggression toward good internal objects (Klein 1948), the country of origin being one of them. Hostile wishes and fantasies involving it therefore must be brought out in the open. Only then can deeper sadness emerge and genuine substitutes for lost objects be found.

Interpreting Defensive Functions of Nostalgia as well as Defenses against the Emergence of Nostalgia

When it comes to the experience of nostalgia, technical interventions with the immigrant and the exile vary considerably. This should not be surprising since the two have very different experiences in this regard. The immigrant is immensely prone to idealizing his country of origin and the exile feels the opposite (see Chapter 3). The analyst should be prepared for much nostalgic rumination in the treatment of the former and little in the treatment of the latter.

The therapist must empathize with the immigrant's loss of historical continuity and the need for its restoration. Patients' lapses into nostalgia must find respect and empathic counterresonance in the analyst. The therapist, however, must not overlook the fact that nostalgic yearning can be used as a psychic ointment to soothe frustration and rage in the external reality as well as in the transference.

Case 5

A Peruvian woman in analysis began talking about her beloved grandmother's funeral some years ago, almost immediately after I had told her of my unavailability for a few days. The connection was obvious. I waited. Gradually, intricate details of Peruvian funeral rituals began to occupy her associations. Her momentary sadness upon my telling her that I would not be available for three days was now replaced with a vigorous tone. I too found myself raptly absorbed in the material, feeling enriched by learning all the cultural details. Returning to a self-observing stance a few minutes later, I noted that she not only had defensively warded off her pain but also had given me a parting gift, as it were. Interpretive interventions along this line deepened the material and facilitated

the analysis of her disappointment at my being away and her subsequent anger about it.

Expression of warm feelings about things "back home" can also
be a shy deflection of acknowledging the pleasure of belonging in
the here and now of the analyst's office.

Case 6

A somewhat schizoid and narcissistic young man from Italy was
in analysis in the United States with an analyst who was clearly not
of Italian extraction. A long "cocoon phase" (Modell 1976) of
narcissistic withdrawal, during which the patient went on and on
about the beauty of his motherland, characterized the beginning
of the analysis. Gradually, as a result of the analyst's holding and
interpreting activities, this phase came to an end. Around this time
the patient began to shyly express his fondness of the analyst's
office. He was especially vivid about it toward the end of one session. However, he started the next hour by reverting to recount-
ing the glory of Italy and the depth of his longing to return to the
country of his origin. The defensive function of such nostalgia
against the acknowledgment of the libidinal gratification of feeling "at home" in the analyst's office (and with the analyst) was clear,
and an interpretation of this led to further deepening of the transference material.

The contemporary emphasis that the immigrant places upon his
nostalgic yearning must not make one overlook that the sentiment
attributed to the loss of one's homeland might have its basis in an
incomplete mourning of a disrupted early mother–child relationship. Sterba (1934) was the first to correlate "homesickness" with
a longing for the maternal breast. Fenichel (1945) also explained
nostalgia as a wish to return to the preoedipal mother. Fodor (1950)
went so far as to trace nostalgic yearnings to a deep-seated longing
for the undisturbed prenatal state. The elegance of these formulations notwithstanding, Hartmann's (1964) warning regarding the
genetic fallacy must be heeded here. In other words, references to

prenatal bliss, maternal breast, and preoedipal mother, in this context, should be viewed as largely metaphorical. Combining this caution with a healthy skepticism toward the literalness of the immigrant's current suffering yields a resilient technique that views the lament of contemporary dislocation and the wailing about childhood loss as defending against each other in a dialectical fashion.

Work with refugees and exiles, however, requires a different technical approach. Instead of allowing psychic space for the elaboration of losses, empathizing with the attendant pain, and analyzing its defensive functions, the analyst has to deal with an individual who does not miss his country of origin at all. Because such an individual is almost invariably deeply traumatized, the analyst's task, for a long time, remains centered upon empathizing with how *bad*, and not how good, the country that has been left indeed was. As this work proceeds, the patient may unwittingly begin to reveal the existence of some pleasant memories of the homeland as well. The analyst, however, must not bring these to the patient's attention too quickly; that would only lead to a defensive recoil. After a sufficient length of time and with the security that his complaints are regarded as legitimate—as they indeed often are—the patient might be prepared to bring into his full consciousness the opposite constellation of his attitude.[51] To undo the psychic compartmentalization caused by splitting thus necessitates that the analyst retain the patient's contradictory emotional attitudes in mind and make "bridging interventions" (Akhtar 1998a, Kernberg 1975, p. 96) that gently demonstrate their coexistence to the patient. Indeed, the analyst must also analyze the defenses against the emergence of nostalgic longing. He must demonstrate to the patient that the catastrophe that forced him out of his homeland also rendered him unable to recall anything positive about his homeland,

---

51. In a study of 1,348 Southeast Asian refugees resettled in Vancouver, British Columbia, Beiser and Hyman (1997) found it was only when the safety and predictability of a routine life were restored that these survivors of adversity permitted the past to emerge into consciousness and began to experience nostalgia.

as the trauma spread backward to poison the good times before it. In other words, (1) empathy with the "bitter" side of the patient's negative nostalgia, (2) interpretive resolution of the defenses against nostalgia, and (3) bridging interventions to link up the sweet with the bitter memories of the homeland are the three mainstays of the analytic treatment of refugees and exiles.

In sum, whether it is the "privacy of the self" (Khan 1983) or the theater of the analytic discourse, the immigrant *and* the exile both struggle with defensive alterations of libidinal investment in the memory of their homeland (and its inevitable linkage to the early maternal imago). The immigrant needs to exaggerate the love that the exile is compelled to deny. By helping the former renounce such idealization and the latter to reclaim the warded-off good feelings, the analyst facilitates genuine affection for the country of origin in both types of individuals. And it is only with such foundation that true commitment to the country of adoption, where life is now to be lived, becomes possible.

Accepting Seemingly Inoptimal Individuation and Involvement of Relatives in Treatment

Writing in a context totally different from the one under consideration here, Searles (1977) observed[52] that "Some patients' reminiscences about childhood are expressed not in terms of 'I,' but rather in terms of 'we.' Such a patient almost invariably recalls that 'we' used to do this and that. He scarcely ever says 'I' in this connection. . . . My impression is that the patient's sense of identity is essentially symbiotic in nature" (p. 444).

Similar psychic constellations of the self-structure have been reported in non-Western patients. Kakar (1985), writing of Indian patients, states that "the relational orientation is still the 'natural'

---

52. Because Searles was not writing about non-Western patients, the phenomena of enmeshed and symbiotic identity would seem to be independent of culture. At the same time, this does not rule out the possibility that such identity may be modal in some cultures and an "outlying" phenomenon in others.

way of viewing the self and the world. Thus it is not uncommon for family members, who often (and significantly!) accompany the patient for a first interview, to complain about the patient's autonomy as one of the symptoms of his disorder" (p. 446).

Roland (1988), having worked with Indian and Japanese patients in their respective countries as well as in the United States, has coined the phrase "familial self" for their central psychic structure. According to him, the degree of psychic separateness and of firmness of self-boundaries is much greater in the United States than it is in India and Japan[53] (see also Yamamoto and Wagatsuma 1980). In the latter societies, the developing self stays forever in emotionally close and interdependent relationships. The individual retains a constant need for approval from others for his self regard. Separation and individuation, conceptualized as intertwined tracks by Mahler and Furer (1968), are farther apart from each other than they are in the West. In other words, the non-Western self can achieve high degrees of individuation without comparable achievement of separateness.

Echoing a similar sentiment, Bonovitz (1998) raises the intriguing question: "If Mahler had emigrated to India rather than the United States, what theory of separation-individuation would she have woven from observations of Indian mothers and their babies?" (p. 178). Bonovitz carefully reviews the pertinent literature and concludes that in many non-Western patients

> Infantile objects are relinquished very gradually, and this process does not take place to the degree necessary in cultures where the child is being prepared to live an adult life that is independent of the extended family. Indian immigrants to the United States are thus transplanted into a very different cultural milieu that emphasizes autonomy and self-sufficiency rather than interdependence. [p. 182]

---

53. Roland (1988 1996) also makes significant distinctions between the Indians and Japanese. Indians, in his opinion, are less secretive and much more in touch with their inner world than the Japanese. The latter have a "far more perfectionistic ego ideal and rigorous social etiquette than Indians" (Roland 1996, p. 19).

There are four clinical consequences of the patient's having such enmeshed identity or familial self. *First,* the treatment of an adult patient might also involve his or her relatives. The analyst might have to make occasional and judicious concessions to the therapeutic framework in this regard. He may have to meet the family members, at least in the beginning of treatment, and, at times, even once or twice during ongoing treatment. Otherwise, the treatment might be put into serious jeopardy (see Case 8, p. 146).

Second, the analyst might have to peacefully accept the greater than customary concern that his adult patient displays for his parents while making important life decisions. While certainly not losing sight of reaction formations pervasive in this realm, such involvement must not be automatically deemed pathological.

Third, in the treatment of patients who come from cultures in which a familial self is the modal psychic structure, the analyst is often faced with multiple transferences (including those involving extrafamilial figures) and a profusion of close and distant relatives in the associative material. Taketomo's (1989) observations regarding the Japanese patient's "teacher transference" (the elementary school teacher, usually a male, is the first truly nonmaternal object in Japan) are significant in this context.

Finally, the seemingly inoptimal capacity for psychic separateness would inevitably affect the patient's relationship with the analyst as well. Advice seeking, need for contact during prolonged separations, prolongation of the termination phase, and, occasionally, a need for predetermined post-termination contacts (Schachter et al. 1997), or at least an explicit "permission" for post-termination contact are various technical accompaniments of such "inoptimal" individuation. Mehta's (1997) giving a "five-minute warning" (p. 464) before the end of the session to her Indian immigrant patients also belongs in this category.

Facing the Challenge Posed by the Patient's Polyglottism and Polylingualism

While Freud privately noted that he found conducting analysis in English "strenuous" (Gay 1988, p. 389), his professional writings regarding language remained restricted to the elucidation of unconscious verbal bridges in the formation of dreams and jokes (Freud 1900, 1905). He did not confront the specific issue of polylingualism in the clinical situation from a theoretical or technical perspective.

It was Ferenczi who first paid attention to this matter. In a paper entitled "Obscene Words," Ferenczi (1911) gave the example of a patient who used euphemisms and foreign words to avoid saying "fart." This suggests that certain words (e.g., obscene words, curses, words for genitals and sex acts) have a greater emotional valence in an individual's mother tongue than in a later acquired language. In the later language, speaking such words is associated neither with a comparable id-discharge nor a strong superego retribution. Ferenczi suggested that obscene words, in their very utterance, approximate the action they are intended to describe. Such thought–action closeness gives them their discharge potential and communicative power. This opens up the clinically significant possibility that polylingual patients

> have at their disposal a defense that allows them to avoid areas in their psychic life that are problematic. By changing language, they will be able to avoid not only the subset, but the whole language of infantile sexuality, thus denying themselves and us access to an area so intimately linked to specific verbal sounds and special names. [Amati-Mehler et al. 1993, p. 34]

The issue of polylingualism in the clinical situation goes beyond obscene words. Using one language as against the other, a polylingual patient can avoid a whole set of traumatic events and memories. Greenson (1950), for instance, reports the treatment of a bilingual German/English woman. At one point the patient refused to speak in German saying, "I have a feeling that talking in German I shall have to remember something I want to forget" (p. 19). Freud's lapsing into Latin, *matrem nudam*, while describing at age 41 the childhood memory of having seen his mother naked is another striking example of defensive use of a second language (letter to Fliess, October 3, 1897, in Masson 1985, p. 268).

Moreover, a word is not merely a denotative agent. It is an element that, by inserting itself into the chain of associations, can modify an entire network of ideas. While the resulting differences are more marked in polylingual patients, the same effect can crop up in monolingual patients using different words for the same thing. Take, for instance, the difference between saying "oral sex" and saying "blow job." Or note the fact that what in North America is called a "flashlight" is called a "torch" all across the English-speaking British commonwealth. Clearly, the two words each have a different aesthetic and sensual feel to them and give rise to different verbal and visual associations.

Another area in which the polylingualism of a patient can pose technical challenges as in the expression of feelings. Not all terms for affect states are readily translatable from one language into another. For instance, the Japanese *amae* finds a poor substitute in the English "affection." The English word "amused" has no counterpart in Urdu. To be sure, many other examples can be readily given. Filet (1998), an immigrant psychoanalyst practicing in Amsterdam, notes that

> Latin ways of expressing experience are often different from Anglo-Saxon, or Germanic ones, making it even harder to estimate [their] semantics. Latin languages often prefer conceptually abstract substantive forms where the other languages would use active forms forgoing nouns. I used to get a bit worried about the quality of the affective experience when I heard Spanish or Portuguese patients say things like: "the jealousy of the other produced inhibition in me," "my pity is no match for my hatred," or "the overcoming of my disillusion renders me stupefied." Whereas a Dutch patient might have said (the Dutch equivalent of): "I was so disappointed that at first I couldn't think of anything." Only gradually have I understood that the use of nouns with an ideational root as opposed to the use of verbs with an action root does not, per se, in persons with dissimilar cultural and linguistic backgrounds, imply different affective intensities or qualities. [pp. 41–42]

Finally, language, having developed as a relational bridge between the self and the other, contains within itself "both the verbal symbols and the representation of the primary 'other' who offered those symbols" (Pérez Foster 1996, p. 248). From this perspective, linguistic shifts of a polylingual patient can be seen as also shifting the specific aspect of the self that is speaking as well as the person who is being spoken to. In essence, from all five perspectives, namely (1) repression of infantile sexuality, (2) avoidance of traumatic events and memories, (3) impact on the associative network, (4) recognition of affects, and (5) oscillation of self- and object representations, linguistic shifts in the clinical situation are highly important.

While this is well accepted, the way in which such shifts are to be technically handled seems far from settled. Some analysts (Buxbaum 1949, Greenson 1950) require that the patient speak, or at least utter some significant words, in his mother tongue. In taking this position, they are not only bowing to Ferenczi's (1911) terse reminder regarding the greater emotional valence of obscene words in the mother tongue, but also asserting that verbalizing experiences in the language in which they took place makes them more vivid, more alive, and hence more useful for treatment purposes. (See also Karpf [1935] in this connection.)

Other analysts, including Lagache (1956), Bennani (1985), who conducts analyses in both Arabic and French, and Amati-Mehler and colleagues (1993), hold a different opinion. They argue that actively encouraging the patient to speak in his mother tongue has the risk of "nourishing the narcissistic illusion of 'total communication'" (Amati-Mehler et al. 1993, p. 81). They recommend that the analyst be more interested in the defensive uses of the second language, the forces underlying the emergence of a wish to speak in one's mother tongue, the rigid and apprehensive avoidance of the mother tongue, the meaning of wanting an analyst who does or does not speak one's mother tongue, and, in essence, the dynamic "moment when the analytic relationship reconfronts the themes linked to the mother tongue" (Amati-Mehler et al. 1993, p. 80). Viewed in this fashion, technical choices regarding language must derive not from rigid formulas but from the specific ebb and flow of the analytic material and the emotional ambience both of the relationship and of the particular session. One should neither encourage nor discourage the patient's use of his mother tongue. And, when the patient appears to be warding off the use of his mother tongue, one should address the reasons for such defensive repudiation.

Case 7

A 34-year-old Pakistani pharmacologist, whose mother tongue was Urdu, was in analysis with an English-speaking North American analyst. One day, during a particular phase of analysis when oedipal transferences were in the forefront of clinical work, the patient suddenly stopped talking. Becoming nervous, he revealed that a word was coming to his mind that he wanted to say but felt he could not utter in the presence of his analyst. The analyst inquired about the imagined danger in speaking the word. "It is just not done. Speaking like that in front of you would be indecent, wrong." Fear of hurting the analyst and being punished in retaliation emerged as the session went on. Toward the end of the session, perhaps drawing a feeling of safety from his approaching exit, the patient finally revealed that the word was *Maader-chod* (literally, motherfucker). The analyst asked the meaning of the word and, upon being told, responded by saying, "Perhaps you were having difficulty in saying this word not only in front of me but to me!" The patient understood the oedipal interpretation and nodded in agreement.

On the other hand, when the patient does talk in his mother tongue (as many immigrant patients do once they feel more or less settled in the treatment situation), the therapist should listen patiently, not rushing the patient to translate the words too quickly. This would allow for the analysis not only of the content but of the feelings (e.g., sadness, triumph), and fantasies associated with speaking a language different than that of the analyst.

SUMMARY

One must distinguish the acquisition of knowledge,
which comes about as a result of modification of pain

(then the knowledge obtained will be used for new
discoveries), from possession of knowledge, which is
used to avoid painful experiences. [Grinberg and
Grinberg 1989, pp. 65–66]

After briefly commenting upon whether psychoanalysis and psychoanalytic psychotherapy are applicable to non-Western, immigrant patients, I have argued that indeed these treatment modalities are useful for this clinical population. I have then outlined eight technical guidelines for such work. These include (1) developing and maintaining cultural neutrality, (2) respecting cultural differences in the experience of time and in the degrees of deference, (3) adopting a developmental stance and conducting developmental work, (4) helping the patient disengage cultural from intrapsychic conflicts, (5) validating feelings of dislocation and facilitating mourning, (6) interpreting defensive functions of nostalgia as well as defenses against the emergence of nostalgia, (7) accepting seemingly inoptimal individuation and involvement of relatives, and (8) facing the challenge posed by the patient's polyglottism and polylingualism. I have emphasized that these are only guidelines and not rules. In psychologically minded and more individuated patients where the treatment method can approach psychoanalysis proper their use recedes to the background. In less sophisticated patients with symbiotic identities and a marked propensity toward cultural rationalizations, these guidelines demand greater attention. In this connection, it should also be remembered that many immigrant patients actually fall in the second category, a group that stands to benefit more from family- and community-oriented approaches.

THE IMMIGRANT COMMUNITY AND THE IMMIGRANT THERAPIST

The guidelines discussed in the preceding chapter pertain largely to adult immigrants seeking psychotherapy and psychoanalysis. These guidelines can be easily tailored to fit child and family interventions of relatively customary types. However, implicit once again is a certain selectivity of sample since only the more educated and psychologically sophisticated among the immigrant population seek such help. Though they do suffer from a variety of conflicts on intrapsychic and interpersonal fronts, the majority of them do not. Rather than turning one's back on these immigrants, the profession needs to (1) make an effort to understand their resistances to seeking help, (2) reach out to them with psycho-educative efforts, (3) offer help in innovative ways, and (4) attempt to recruit more members of the immigrant groups to the mental health professions ranging from social work through psychiatry and clinical psychology to psychoanalysis.

One area of "immediacy," to borrow a phrase used by Strachey (1934) in a different context, in all immigrant groups is that of parent–child communication. Interventions at this level always seem needed and attempts to open up a dialogue with immigrant families are seldom unwelcome.

CHILD AND FAMILY INTERVENTIONS

> Anxious about their diminished authority, some [im-
> migrant] grandparents and parents resort to auto-
> cratic rule, scapegoating of more vulnerable mem-
> bers (such as the elderly, the less functional, or a
> spouse), and revisiting of outside influences. [Cook
> and Timberlake 1989, p. 91]

> Puerto Rican adolescents not only have to contend
> with the developmental difficulties of this growth
> period, but also with factors related to their status
> either as a recent immigrant, as a first-, second-, or
> third-generation Puerto Rican, or as an *entremundos*
> youth. [Martinez 1994, p. 98, original italics]

Immigrant parents—whether they are from India, South Korea, Puerto Rico, China, Mexico, or Iran—are involved in a lifelong mourning process. At each step in their lives they are reminded that the ego etiquette by which they would have lived is no more their guide. Speaking a later acquired language, "barred from weddings and funerals" (Akhtar 1995a, p. 1077), continually try-ing to learn proper manners for age-appropriate social occasions, immigrant parents have burdened egos. This, coupled with their having little help from the community or extended family, might make them encourage their children to be quite autonomous at a very young age. In less culturally informed settings, imitation of the supposedly Western modes of child-rearing might also fuel such a tendency.

All this, however, comes down crashing once their offspring reach adolescence. This is the time when children exert their au-tonomy, rebel, and need to individuate from parents. Even non-immigrant parents are taxed by the regressive and progressive vac-illations of their adolescent children. This burden is greater for immigrant parents. Having compromised their psychohistorical links with their own earlier generations, immigrant parents expe-rience the needed letting-go of the child as losing him or her. Matters are made more complex because of the bicultural idiom of the battles surrounding the adolescent's assertion of selfhood.

Parental lack of comprehension in this regard ("Dating is not fucking, Mom!" yelled a 16-year-old daughter of immigrant Iranian parents) compounds the pain of "losing" a child. The last-ditch hope of retaining unchanged links to one's culture of origin is threatened and deepens parents' anguish. This is paralleled by the challenges faced by the adolescent who is born in the country of adoption.

> A child who is raised without much of her parents' original culture can feel a huge separation and detachment from the parents as well as from their country of origin. Such a child does not understand certain essential ways of her parents, which were defined by the parents' culture (e.g., issues involving respect, nuances of language). This might result in conflicts between the youth and parents that can last until that cultural gap is somehow bridged.
>
> If children grow up in a country where their physical attributes (color of skin, facial characteristics, etc.) render them a distinct minority, *and* they do not have a strong sense of belonging to their parents' country of origin, their identity can become fractured. Matters become worse if, in school, they are confronted with the issue through teasing by peers. They have neither a rationale as to why they look a certain way nor a satisfactory retaliation to the prejudiced and irrational banter of others. [Nishat Akhtar, personal communication, June 1999]

Having been exposed to a greater than ordinary difference between the family culture and the culture at large, the first-generation adolescent is faced by a double burden (Martinez 1994, Mehta 1998, Phinney et al. 1990). On the one hand, his task is to establish a secure beginning of young adulthood (sexual identity and experience, vocational choice, and increased psychic separateness) and, in the process, move away from his parents. On the other, he is often ill-equipped for the cultural exigencies of the reality outside the home. While he needs to disengage from the parental ethos and find his own way of negotiating life's challenges, he is burdened with the cultural vulnerability of his immigrant parents and hence feels inhibited in rebelling against them. He feels too assimilated vis-à-vis the culture at large with respect to his parents, but he is regarded as too ethnic by his peers. And despite a longing for disengagement from the ethnic culture, there is the longing for it.[54] Tara Ramchandani, the 16-year-old daughter of an Indian American friend, gives voice to this latter sentiment in her 1998 poem, "Past Voices":

> An ocean away past voices
> Beckoning with promises of rickshaws, bindis and saris.
> Part of my soul inside unknown.
> I yearn to know more,
> To be brimming, spilling over
> With brown friends who look like me.
> Words like chapati and Om.
> Waiting to be found and claimed.

When such yearning is truly intense, however, the issue is most likely not a cultural one. A desperate search for ethnicity almost always suggests hunger for parental—especially maternal—acceptance and love, with such acceptance often acting as a balm against unconscious guilt involving hostile and incestuous fantasies. This is what I would term as the *law of suspicious cultural intensity*. In other words, mild cultural hunger is cultural, while more intense forms of it are the result of deeper unresolved conflicts. Of course, the first-generation immigrant adolescent has additional pressures upon him. The disharmonious and conflicting values of one's parents and one's peers put an extra burden upon the adolescent's ego, rendering identity consolidation difficult.[55] Such a child has to create

> a "third reality," neither of his or her parents' homeland nor of the adopted land, but uniquely and historically different. . . . This third

---

54. At times a temporary solution is to find an identity that is neither ethnic nor assimilated; Tang (1992) has described four cases of Chinese American young women who temporarily chose to adopt European identities instead of either Chinese or American identities.

55. Even more difficult, perhaps, is the situation of the adolescent who has just arrived as a migrant in a new country (see Chapter 1).

space spans the inner and outer reality. Social role is affected by events within the social cultural context to which the ego must adapt, such as the conflicting reality . . . [an] adolescent is faced with, and the rapidly shifting cultures, ethnic and monoethnic, within the home and outside. . . . constantly changing and diffusely defined roles place a certain stress on the ego and could decisively compromise its identifications. [Mehta 1998, p. 137]

Two problematic outcomes are the development of ethnocentric and alienated identities. In the former, the child remains comfortable at home and in homoethnic groups but finds it difficult to mingle with the culture at large. In the latter, the child feels comfortable neither at home nor in the world outside it. Both types of children are prone (the latter more so than the former) to considerable psychosocial turmoil during adolescence. Such adolescents and their families need help. Under fortunate circumstances, either psychoanalysis proper or individual psychotherapy is sought and can be provided. However, focus on individual treatment must not minimize the importance of parallel work with parents. In this connection, Mehta's (1998) delineation of the difficulties that might arise when immigrant parents seek therapists of their own background is highly pertinent. "A common rescue fantasy is elicited based on a pseudo-bond of one immigrant helping another in a foreign country. . . . However there is also a rapid fantasy formation of parents' having control over the (immigrant) therapist, and fear that an American therapist will be intimidating and will not comply with their wishes" (p. 150).

Keeping such pitfalls in mind while retaining empathy for the parents who are themselves feeling wounded and vulnerable would lead to a therapeutic stance that is optimally interpretive and supportive of them (Prathikanti 1997, Tummala 1998). The need for family interventions might, however, extend beyond the usual age group considered adolescent. Sometimes, even in the course of adult psychotherapy and psychoanalysis, judicious contact with the patient's family might be necessary and useful.

Case 8

A 24-year-old South-Indian Brahmin woman sought help for her anguished love life. Having arrived in the United States at age 4, she had grown up in a relatively conservative immigrant Hindu family living in a large East Coast city. Finishing high school with accolades, she entered an Ivy League university and did extremely well there. After that she got a job, postponing further studies for later.

The problem for which she ostensibly sought help was basically this: she was deeply in love with an African American man (who had been a college classmate of hers) but her parents had raised hell about it. Her father was constantly yelling and screaming at her on the phone. Her mother was having "a heart attack, every day." A huge amount of shame and guilt was inflicted upon her. She was repeatedly told (often in phone calls made to her at her workplace) that she had brought shame to the family, indeed to the entire Indian immigrant community in the parental town. She was given the damning choice of staying involved with her boyfriend or retaining ties with her family.

In the first few interviews, it became clear that the problem was much more complex. Conflict existed at three levels in the interpersonal realm: (1) the clash between her liberal disposition and the post-colonial racist attitude of her parents, (2) the antagonism between Indian immigrant parents with a "familial self" (Roland 1988) as their main psychic structure and the more individuated and autonomous decision-making process of their acculturated daughter who had grown up in the United States, and, (3) an ordinary intergenerational conflict that could have occurred in a nonimmigrant setting also, if the parents strongly disapproved of the mate chosen by their child.

Lying deeper than these interpersonal scenarios was the intrapsychic conflict of the patient who, as it turned out, had been extremely close to her father and at age 8 or so had been sexually abused by an uncle of hers; attempts she made to convey this to her parents went unheard. So in the intrapsychic realm too, two levels of conflict seemed to exist (1) a powerful oedipal fixation, and (2) much unresolved shame about childhood incestuous abuse and rage at her parents, especially her mother, for not having rescued her. The patient's choice of the "unacceptable" African American boyfriend now appeared as a disguise for the prohibited father as well as a retaliation toward both parents for not having saved her from the uncle.

The inflammable mixture of these five levels of conflict posed a true therapeutic challenge. The situation was compounded by constant harassment of the patient by her parents. This flooded her ego with so much panic that little in the form of psychotherapy could be done. When I suggested to her that she encourage her family to seek therapy or even that her parents seek help simply to manage their turmoil, I learned that they would not go to anyone. However, since they knew that I was a fellow immigrant from India, they conveyed their willingness to meet with me. Bending the frame of therapy, I agreed to conduct a few family meetings. It was only with this maneuver that some calm was achieved, boundaries drawn, and beginning of deeper treatment of the patient made possible.

Such family interventions in a 24-year-old individual who is living on her own are not in the usual armamentarium of an analyst. If the analyst can manage to have both flexibility of perspective and a tempered yet deep regard for the spirit over the letter of the analytic rules and guidelines, he will be able to come up with what is technically needed.

PSYCHOANALYTICALLY INFORMED ADVICE

> I arranged with Hans's father that he should tell the boy that all this business about horses was a piece of nonsense and nothing more. The truth was, his father was to say, that he was very fond of his mother and wanted to be taken into her bed. The reason he was afraid of horses now was that he had taken so much interest in their widdlers. [Freud 1909, p. 28]

> advice: 1: recommendation regarding a decision or
> course of conduct . . . ; 2: information or notice
> given . . . ; 3: an official notice concerning a busi-
> ness transaction. [*Merriam-Webster's Collegiate Dictio-
> nary* 1987, p. 59]

Yet another unusual form of intervention is what I have come to call *psychoanalytically informed advice.* This might appear a bit of an oxymoron at first sight since, as analysts, we are always in awe of the complex and multiple determinants (Waelder 1936) of human behavior. Hence, we view advice as essentially useless and even risky. At best, it is ineffective. At worst, it transiently tilts the balance of a conflict in one direction at the sacrifice of deeper elucidation of its various unconscious ramifications. Holding this to be true of clinical psychoanalysis and psychotherapy, I have nevertheless come to believe that some situations exist where an analyst might indeed offer informed advice.[56] Certain conditions must, however, exist for this. The following two cases might illustrate what I have in mind.

Case 9

A young mother with a 7-year-old son and a 5-year-old daughter reported an intriguing behavior on the part of her daughter. Fond of a family friend of theirs, the little girl initiated a game that she called "blind animals" with him. This family friend would draw the picture of an animal (e.g., elephant, turtle, owl) and she would gleefully scribble out the animal's eyes, bursting into laughter and saying that "this animal is blind."

When her mother asked me why the girl did this, I suggested that perhaps she was seeing something that she did not want to see. As we talked along these lines, I became reasonably certain that the girl was not witnessing the primal scene. Yet I felt that she was indeed exposed to something that was producing anxiety. I persisted in my inquiry and it turned out to be fruitful. The mother

---

56. Freud's (1909) treatment of Little Hans, largely conducted via the boy's father, is an example par excellence of such an intervention.

bathed the two naked children together in the tub every day, exposing the little girl to her older brother's genitals. As we discussed its potential impact on the little girl, I advised the mother to put an end to this practice. While a bit incredulous, the mother decided to do what I had told her. When I met her a few weeks later, I was told that the little girl had completely lost interest in playing the "blind animals" game with the family friend!

While other determinants might have played a role, it seems clear to me that my advice to her mother protected the little girl from the anxiety-producing vision of her brother's genitals. Her anxiety diminished and so did the need to play the "blind animals" game.

The second case (Akhtar 1999e) also demonstrates the usefulness of such counsel, although the context and interventions used were quite different.

Case 10

While visiting Bombay a few years ago, I was approached by a wealthy young woman in the middle of a cocktail party. While she seemed to know me, I had some difficulty in recognizing her at first. The reasons for this soon became clear. I had met her and her husband a few years before in London where they used to live and work. I learned that they had migrated back to India and were thoroughly enjoying themselves. The reason I had difficulty recognizing her, however, was not totally due to this time gap. She had changed her appearance considerably and was completely decked out in gorgeous traditional Indian attire. Sari, red dot on forehead, the works!

She said that she and her husband needed my help since they were very worried about their young child. This, too, was news to me. Apparently, they had had a child, a son who was then about 3 years old. We arranged a meeting for the following day.[57]

---

57. In the past, I would decline requests for consultations made during parties in India. More recently, I have changed my mind, thinking that well-informed advice might either not be sought otherwise or might actually not be available.

The next day, she came with her husband, a solid, and, generally speaking, a well-meaning man. She was dressed in elegant Indian attire. As we talked, I learned that their son had regressed after their arrival in India, two months earlier. His physical health was fine but his behavior had changed for the worse. He would scream, refuse to go to sleep, cling, and, at times, spit on people. From their descriptions, the child appeared angry, while his parents seemed thrilled about returning to their motherland.

I suspected that the child was responding to the parental shift of attention (they were busy relocating and enjoying themselves), loss of the familiar visual and sonic surround of England, and, above all, "loss" of the mother he was familiar with—she looked so different. I asked her about her dressing habits and she proudly told me that she had completely Indianized her wardrobe and changed her appearance.

Upon listening to all this, I suggested that the mother restrict wearing Indian clothes to evening parties, at least for the next six months or so. I explained to her that if I had difficulty recognizing her, how must her little boy feel about this sartorial inconstancy? I also recommended that they hire as fair-complexioned a house staff as possible and plaster the child's bedroom walls with pictures of his room in their London house and of his British babysitters. Through these maneuvers, I was attempting to create a "British" holding environment for the child. The parents, intelligent as they were, asked if all this would not make it harder for the boy to "leave" England. I said "No, this will put it under his control. He will walk out to India in the living room and walk back to England in his room.[58] This will give him control over the trauma of loss and ease his suffering." I also told the couple that while I

---

58. In effect, I was trying to create an environmental "fort-da" (Freud 1920). For those unfamiliar with the notion, the phrase refers to an 18-month-old child's utterance while throwing a wooden reel out of his crib and delightfully retrieving it by pulling at the string. Freud, who silently observed the child (actually his grandson) regarded this play as the child's attempt to master separation from his mother.

was returning to the States, they should call me on a monthly basis and give me an update on how things were going.

The results of this consultation turned out to be highly gratifying. The child quickly bounced back to his usually ebullient self. While it is certainly possible that my psychoanalytically informed advice worked in ways other than I intended, it surely was far from ineffective!

The common elements in these two instances are (1) diminished likelihood of seeking (Case 9) or actual unavailability (Case 10) of psychoanalytic help, (2) the symptomatic individual being a child, (3) symptomatology of short duration and of mild to moderate severity, and (4) concerned and inquisitive parents. That unsolicited advice, psychoanalytically informed or otherwise is not to be given goes without saying.

COMMUNITY OUTREACH

> The Vietnamese communities that have emerged as part of the secondary migration and as part of the support systems of refugee families today represent untapped potential. They provide a means for maintaining the Vietnamese refugees' cultural heritage as well as a means for building bridges with the multicultural American heritage. [Cook and Timberlake 1989, p. 96]

> Communities provide important social support. In the absence of ethnic communities, pseudo-communities may help. However, sponsors, hosts, and others involved in creating a welcome for newcomers require backup and help to be effective in bridging cultural gaps. [Beiser 1990, p. 62]

Psycho-educative workshops for immigrant families and children allow the therapist ready access to subterranean emotional problems in this group. Community outreach activities thus acquire a great significance. Workshops involving adolescents and their parents, at first separately and then together, might beneficially address issues of identity, dating, sexual behavior, vocational choices, and the necessary separateness and autonomy of growing children from their parents.

The highly sophisticated work of the Nafsiyat Intercultural Therapy Centre with minority and immigrant populations in England (Kareem and Littlewood 1992, Littlewood 1992a,b); the long-standing multipronged approach of the Dutch Organization for the Mental Health of Immigrants and Refugees in Amsterdam (PHAROS) (van Essen 1999); the highly meaningful school-level interventions by the Canadian Task Force on Mental Health Issues Affecting Immigrants and Refugees; and the counseling and psycho-educational efforts of Connections, a cross-cultural foster-care agency in Falls Church, Virginia, which specializes in dealing with Southeast Asian refugees (Hunt 1989), are some outstanding examples of such community oriented efforts.

Within psychoanalytic organizations proper, such outward effort is just beginning. The American Psychoanalytic Association established the Ad-Hoc Committee on Racial and Ethnic Diversity in 1994, a task-oriented group that has now become a standing committee of the organization. This committee has been assigned the task of encouraging greater minority representation on the various scientific programs of the American Psychoanalytic Association, preparing model bibliographies and curricula regarding psychoanalysis and cultural diversity, organizing scientific programs at local and national levels, exploring ways and means of encouraging minority candidate recruitment, and bringing together the various community outreach programs already in existence at the various institutes and societies of the American Psychoanalytic Association. The International Psychoanalytic Association has also undertaken a similar sort of mission on a worldwide scale. Its newly formed Committee for Development of Psychoanalysis in Asia, for instance, has been assigned the task of assessing the status of the few existing (and often moribund) psychoanalytic societies in Asian countries and of seeking ways to propagate psychoanalytic knowledge in these nations, especially by supporting the interest groups that have newly arisen there.

Finally, the movement toward cultural pluralism and communal inclusiveness is also discernible at a grass-roots level in the component societies and institutes of the American Psychoanalytic Association. While some centers, for example Michigan (Mehta 1995), are much more active than others, most societies and institutes of the American Psychoanalytic Association are beginning to undertake some form of community outreach programs. Efforts are underway to establish liaison between psychoanalytic societies and local schools, universities, day-care centers, art museums, and ethnic organizations. Psychoanalysts are beginning to go out in the community and hold workshops and discussion groups with lay people on topics ranging from day care to divorce, movies to motherhood, and prejudice to poetry. The hope of all such interventions is to increase knowledge of psychological processes in the immigrant populations. This, in turn, can encourage their seeking help and prevent more serious regressions and conflicts. Recruiting more workers in the mental health field from the immigrant groups is another agenda of such outreach activities.

THE IMMIGRANT THERAPIST

> Not prone to taking things for granted and not sharing cultural blind-spots, the immigrant therapist has a greater objectivity in looking at his client's problems. He may indeed have special assets imparted to him by his particular cultural background. Thus, the Latin American medical graduate's exceptional ease in developing an empathic relationship and the Iranian medical graduate's great perceptiveness of nonverbal communication and his "silence tolerance" have been commented upon. [Teja and Akhtar 1981, p. 334]

> The emphasis on analytic communication through words is counter to the dominant Indian idiom in which words are only a small part of a vast store of signs and semiotics. The pitch and intonation of voice, facial expressions, hand gestures and bodily

> movements are expected to play a large role in any
> close interpersonal encounter. These too are expec-
> tations to which the Indian analyst, given his own
> embeddedness in the idiom of the culture, is not
> immune. [Kakar 1985, p. 444]

To be an immigrant and to practice psychotherapy and psychoanalysis largely with native-born patients poses many dilemmas and
challenges. "As a person of color and of a different culture, the
minority therapist is more than just a blank screen, and his or her
color will pull forth a rich variety of projections and stereotypes"
(Tang and Gardner 1999, p. 8). Holmes (1992) refers to the resulting associations as "points of access to a patient's transferences"
(p. 8).

In light of this, the lack of literature on this topic is striking. This
is even more notable in view of the fact that a large number of early
analysts, both in England and the United States, were immigrants.
Perhaps this omission is due to the reluctance of mainstream psychoanalysis to deal with sociological, historical, and cultural factors in adult life in favor of an exclusive focus upon the intrapsychic residues of early childhood.[59] The fact that these European
analysts were actually not immigrants but refugees and exiles might
also have contributed to the profession's silence on this issue.
Wanting to forget their traumatic departures, deny cultural differences with their patients, and become quickly assimilated at a professional level, these analysts did not want to draw others' (and their
own) attention to their ethnic and national origins. Hence they
wrote little about the dilemmas of practicing analysis and psychotherapy as "foreigners."

---

59. Note the skepticism with which the early post-Freudian forays into sociocultural realms (Fromm 1950, Horney 1937, Roheim 1943, 1952) were met by
the profession. Curiously, this attitude did not take into account that Freud
(1921, 1927, 1930, etc.) had a deep and abiding interest in the dialectical relationship between the workings of the individual psyche and the nature of social
institutions. It was as if applied analysis and sociocultural extensions of theory
and technique were deemed only the father's prerogative!

Now the climate is different. Psychoanalysis is undergoing a major cultural rejuvenation.[60] The increase in the number of people migrating from one country to another has resulted in significant shifts in the demographic makeup of the industrialized nations, especially the United States and England. Along with an increase in the culturally diverse patient clientele, there is also an increase in culturally diverse trainees in psychology, social work, psychiatry, and psychoanalysis. The contemporary theoretical pluralism in psychoanalysis is yet another factor that makes it possible, even necessary, to openly discuss technical matters of specific concern to the foreign-born, that is, the "immigrant" therapist.

To begin with, the immigrant analyst should be curious about the patient's choice of analyst. However, asking direct questions in this regard is hardly ever helpful. It can drive the significant material, if it does exist, away from consciousness and behind socially appropriate ego defenses. Also, this gentle skepticism regarding the patient's choice should be tempered by the recognition that, at times, such choices have no "deep" significance at all.[61] At other times, an early and seemingly mundane reference to ethnic matters might be the first hint of major transferences lying in wait.

Case 11

A 40-year-old internist sought consultation with me for some phobic anxieties. He came from a remote suburb and was unfamiliar with downtown Philadelphia. In his first session with me, he said that he was not favorably impressed by the town, and added with a snicker that "too many Vietnamese and Cambodian vendors seem to have moved in here." When I noted the potential allusion

---

60. For a discussion of the academic, organizational, and technical levels of such rejuvenation, see Akhtar (1998b).

61. Only a third of the patients who are in psychotherapy or psychoanalysis with me have revealed significant conscious or unconscious motivations involving my being an immigrant in their choice of me as a therapist.

in this remark to me, the patient quickly denied any ethnic anxieties regarding our working together.[62]

Once the patient was well-settled in analysis, however, he began to display considerable prejudice against Asians. He regarded Indians as being especially incompetent. Still later, he sheepishly revealed that he had deliberately sought an analyst who would be incompetent so that he would not be hurt too much in undergoing analysis. In other words, my expected incompetence would save him from coming to terms with his shame-laden aspects. Projection of his own feelings of being weak and incompetent vis-à-vis his older brother and father gradually was discerned, as were hidden masochistic desires to be hurt and beaten.

While in the beginning an open-minded, patient, and curious attitude is the ideal one to have, the demands made by some patients call for limit setting from the outset. Only then can an investigative collaboration be set in motion.

Case 12

A young Jewish psychologist, whose father was a survivor of the Holocaust, called me seeking psychoanalysis. She was well-informed about analysis and had been given my name by an elderly Jewish training analyst. While setting an appointment on the phone, she asked me: "Are you an Arab?" I responded by saying that while I was interested in her question and what lay behind it, I could not answer it on a factual basis. I added that if we were going to undertake any kind of in-depth work together, my reality was less important than what she made of it in her mind. The patient, however, persisted, saying "Look, I am a devout Jew and an ardent Zionist. I know that if you are an Arab, your sympathies in the Israeli-Palestine conflict will lie with the Palestinians. And I am not about to give my money to someone who will support terrorism against my

---

62. This was many years ago. My manner of asking was perhaps too direct then and might have contributed to his defensive withdrawal.

own people." I was taken aback by the sadomasochistic proclivity I sensed under a thin patina of ethnic rationalization. I responded by repeating what I had said and adding that if she found herself willing to tolerate ambiguity and investigate what had already begun to take place, then perhaps we could meet. Otherwise, she might have to go elsewhere. She came for her appointment and did enter analysis with me.

In the subsequent six years or so, she underwent a rather stormy analysis. Provocative limit-testing and recall through enactments pervaded the early phase. Three things in succession took center stage, though criss-crossing each other: (1) the Holocaust and her contradictory identifications with her father's "survivor's guilt" (Niederland 1968) and his persecutor's sadism, (2) the "separation guilt" (Modell 1984) involving a depressed mother, and (3) a negative oedipal defense against guilt-ridden positive oedipal strivings. These shifts, interestingly, were associated with changing perceptions of my ethnicity: first, an Arab (Nazi), then an Indian Muslim (Jew), and finally, a reasonably assimilated immigrant American.

Such shifting transferences and their corresponding ethnic metaphors[63] warrant that the analyst also scan the associative material for disguised and displaced references to his ethnicity or race (Abbasi 1997, Holmes 1992, Leary 1995). However, this activity should not be done at the cost of sacrificing interest in the deeper meanings of the patient's material. It should also be kept in mind that the patient's every utterance about people of the analyst's ethnicity and race is not transferentially significant. The required tension between skepticism and credulousness might tax the immigrant therapist's ego, especially if he or she is a novice.

---

63. In a paper striking for its clarity and comprehensiveness, Abbasi (1997) describes her (a Muslim analyst's) treatment of an immigrant Jewish patient, offering details not only of the transference–countertransference material, but of her own concurrent analysis, as well as the manner in which this material was handled in her supervision.

Immigrant analysts might also be burdened by the task of maintaining *cultural neutrality* in remaining equidistant from the moral dictates of their own culture and those of the native patients' cultures. While such tension also exists in the native analyst–native patient dyad—because any two individuals can have different moral compasses—its magnitude is potentially greater in the immigrant analyst–native patient dyad.

Yet another area of difficulty might arise if the language in which the immigrant analyst conducts treatment differs from his mother tongue. Obviously, lacking idiomatic fluency in the patient's language, the analyst might occasionally miss puns, witticisms, double entendres, metaphors, and allusions. However, this can also happen in monolingual therapeutic dyads, as there might be linguistic differences based upon regions, subcultures, and social classes. Even an individual family can use words in a way that is idiosyncratic and beyond the empathic grasp of outsiders. While the golden rule is "when in doubt, ask," one hopes that such a need would not arise too frequently and that when it does, it would not be inappropriately inhibited. Asking should not be restricted to clarifying a particular word, but extend to seeking clarification for an abrupt pause in the flow of the patient's speech. Occasionally, this can unmask unexpected anxieties regarding the analyst's ethnicity and, behind them, deeper transference-based concerns.

Case 13

An attractive, midwestern, Catholic lawyer began an analysis with me to overcome her depressive proclivities and enhance her capacity for deeper heterosexual relationships. During a session in the third month of her analysis, she said: "You know, I used to get depressed on Sundays. I felt so lonely. But nowadays, I don't get depressed at all. In fact, if I feel the slightest feeling of gloom coming over me I say to myself that I have . . . ." The patient stopped abruptly in midsentence. After a moment's passage, she finished the sentence by saying ". . . you in my life." Noting the pause, I said:

"What made you pause abruptly? Did you change something in your mind in order to finish the sentence?" The patient then reported that she was about to say that "I say to myself that I have Dr. Akhtar in my life." She explained that she had changed "Dr. Akhtar" to "you," adding that saying it that way seemed more direct to her and made us feel, in her mind, more closely related. I responded "Yes. I can see your point. Yet by changing what was coming to your mind and what you do really say to yourself, you might have created distance between us. I also wonder if there were other reasons leading to your switching the words." The patient then revealed that she had felt anxiety in pronouncing my name. She feared that if she did not pronounce it the "correct" way, that I would regard her as different from me and this would make her feel distant, rejected, and sad. She also wanted to protect me from feeling like a foreigner by bringing attention to my ethnic-sounding name. In essence, neither of us was to feel rejected by the other. Exploration along these lines led to unearthing of lifelong concerns regarding optimal distance and feeling unaccepted in her family of origin.

The mention of the immigrant analyst's ethnic-sounding name brings up the larger topic of his mother tongue. The occasional desire of the immigrant analyst to intervene in his mother tongue (which the patient does not understand) will usually have to be met with ego restraint and further grief work regarding the analyst's own immigration. More importantly, what is needed at such moments is self-analytic inquiry into the specific transaction that triggered such a wish. In other words, the analyst must ask himself or herself the following questions: Why this session? What was in the patient's communication that made me want to respond in my mother tongue? Did the patient's words or feelings touch something deeply personal in me? What? And, in a return to a more objective stance, would conveying the idea that occurred to me be useful to the patient? Or should I just offer a translation? What is the advantage of the former? Would speaking in my mother tongue traumatize the patient or impart genuineness to the relational matrix?

Case 14

A young internist was looking after a hospitalized old man. Both
of them were avid gardeners and often exchanged notes about their
hobby with each other. In her analysis with me, the internist told
me one day that the old man had given her some seeds that she
was planning to plant in her backyard over the weekend. She was
excited since the seeds were for a very rare type of flowering plant.
"Old man," "backyard," "seed," and "flower" clearly constituted
thinly veiled allusions to an oedipal transference fantasy. However,
more important for the context, here is what happened next day.

The patient began sobbing as soon as she entered my office. Her
patient had died the previous night. She cried and said, "What good
are those seeds now? I can't tell him how they fared. Did the flow-
ers come out or not? It's all useless now. I'm just going to throw
the seeds away." Listening to this, I was moved. The urge to say the
following in Urdu came over me: "Sub kahan, khuch laala-o-gul
mein numayan ho gayeen." The line, from the nineteenth-century
doyen of Urdu poetry, Ghalib, is one of the two constituting the
couplet

> Sub kahan, khuch laala-o-gul mein numayan ho gayeen
> khaak mein kya sooraten hongi, jo pinhan ho gayeen.

Roughly translated, these lines mean:

> Not all, only a few of the buried ones emerge as flowers,
> The earth's bosom hides so many faces, talents, and powers.

Given my cultural background, it was the perfect empathic remark
to make.[64] It would have conveyed to the listener that I resonated

---

64. Upon hearing this vignette, a prominent New York analyst said that the
idea of reciting even a single line of poetry in a psychoanalytic session would
appear too pompous and exhibitionistic to him. Clearly, there is a big difference in the intellectual and aesthetic traditions that have formed our child-
hoods—and hence psychostructural backgrounds.

with her pain, helplessness, and sense of loss. However, in the clinical situation, where the patient did not understand my mother tongue, I did not speak the words that had come to my mind. I realized that uttering those words and then translating them would shift her attention from felt pain to intellectual effort; hearing me speak in a different language might cause her intrigue, if not shock. A comment intended to be empathic would thus become just the opposite, a manic defense. So I did not say it. However, in not saying it, I tolerated the helplessness of her not being linguistically "available" to me like the old man was not available to her in reality any more.

At another time, however, I did speak in my mother tongue to a patient who, while multilingual, did not know that particular language.

Case 15

The patient was an intelligent and successful woman in her thirties. Her parents had become divorced when she was 7 years old though she had sensed her father's increasing remoteness for a year or two before that. Following the divorce, the patient felt "invisible" to her father, who paid much more attention to her older sister and brother. The theme of her "invisibility" came up frequently in her analysis and was found to be linked, at its base, to an early maternal depression and a pervasive maternal tendency to invalidate her feelings. It was also related to her father's lack of interest as well as her own defensive retreat from being "visible" to him, since that stirred up all kinds of longings and desires. We worked this through and the patient established a solid romantic partnership with a man. One day she asked me what was the word for "daughter" in my mother tongue. I responded by saying that I was curious about what lay behind her question. Fantasies about my having a daughter emerged. The patient expressed curiosity about how I treated my daughter. Better than her father or the same way? Work along these lines led to our fleshing out further oedipal transference material as well as issues of sibling rivalry (her older sister had been the father's favorite).

However, when in a similar session a few days later she again asked me the Urdu word for "daughter," I responded by saying, "I guess you want to hear the word *Beti* from me not only to satisfy your intellectual curiosity but to see with what feeling tone I say it and also so that I can say it not only in front of you, but as if *to* you." The patient nodded, and began sobbing. I knew that I could have made the same interpretation without the use of the word *Beti*, but felt that her hearing it would provide just the right amount of gratification to her against which further mourning of her father's inattention toward her (and her anger about this) could take place. I am aware that some would argue that this gratification bypassed the analysis of her aggression. I do not agree with that view as there were plenty of other occasions for her discharging and analyzing aggression *and* because I believe that good analytic technique needs optimal and not maximal frustration in order for the patient to remain in an analyzable mode.

These examples of linguistic dilemmas of the immigrant therapist should not make one overlook the fact that similar dilemmas are faced by nonimmigrant therapists too. Defensive alterations of language (e.g., from an instinctually charged word to a sanitized expression) happen in monolingual therapeutic dyads as well. For the immigrant therapist, this becomes strikingly clear when a fellow immigrant from his own linguistic and cultural background enters analysis or psychotherapy with him. The potential for "shared ethnic scotoma" (Shapiro and Pinsker 1973), in which aggression can be displaced onto ethnoculturally or racially different others is increased (Holmes 1992). Other types of countertransference collusions (Tang and Gardner 1999) can also occur,

> especially when the therapist identifies closely with the patient's experiences. The therapist may be more tolerant and less confrontational about some instances of acting out. When this identification is strong, the therapist is often tempted to go the extra mile for the patient. . . . it is a temptation to reach out to such patients, in the sense of being somewhat more didactic and helpful about the process itself. [p. 16]

At the same time, treating patients of his own ethnicity brings an immigrant therapist one big step closer to his native-born colleagues who are exposed to such clinical pitfalls on a daily basis.

All in all, what matters most is the degree to which the immigrant therapist's own mourning over immigration has been successful. His "third individuation" (Akhtar 1995) matters and so does his continuing self-analysis. His ability to maintain cultural neutrality and optimal distance between his own hybrid identity and his patient's relatively monolithic one is of course crucial. Ultimately, however, his deep conviction of the universality of fundamental psychic configurations and the ubiquitousness of human conflicts[65] will help him hear and understand (both within himself and in his patients) "voices that are not necessarily unified and not unifiable" (Amati-Mehler et al. 1993, p. 283) while continuing his analytic work.

SUMMARY

As psychoanalysis is entering its second century, it is timely for us to loosen our preemptory grip on the exclusionary supremacy we have given—and in many corners still maintain—to understanding our patients psychoanalytically solely from our findings in the clinical situation, and to allow explorations of the importance of personality formation and, on the one hand, psychopathology of biology, of genes, and biochemical physiology, and on the other hand, of society, culture, and ethnicity. [Parens 1998, p. 201]

In this chapter, I have highlighted the importance of facilitating the parent–child dialogue through clinical and extraclinical measures. I have emphasized that in certain cultural groups the use of such interventions is not restricted to child patients but

---

65. To be sure, a good experience in one's analysis and clinical supervision goes a long way in establishing this, as do friendships with "natives" that evolve and deepen over a long period of time.

extends to adult patients and their parents. I have also introduced the concept of psychoanalytically informed advice while underscoring that only those with experience might use such an intervention, and then only judiciously. I have also delineated the conditions that justify its use. Following this, I have commented upon the importance of community outreach, for both psycho-educative (hence preventive) and recruitment purposes. I have then devoted a lengthy section to the psychology of the immigrant therapist. In that section, I have underscored the countertransference pitfalls and the linguistic dilemmas of the therapist practicing analysis or psychotherapy far from his original external surround and the home of his internal objects.

As I recount what I have accomplished and approach the end of my book, it is not out of place to acknowledge what I have not been able to include here. My work has focused upon immigrants, their identity problems, and their psychotherapy and psychoanalysis. While I have addressed the problems of exiles, the more acutely devastated refugees, especially in their social and rehabilitative needs, have not received enough attention here.[66] I have also not addressed the more severe end of psychopathology in early immigrants and refugees, including acute paranoid reactions, severe depressions, and suicide (Hovey and King 1996). I acknowledge these limitations and hope that others will pick up where I leave off this work.

At the same time, I feel that by including a large number of conceptual and technical variables, by quoting poems and personal letters, by illustrating clinical issues with examples of both immigrant patients and immigrant analysts, and by bringing sociology, anthropology, literature, psychiatry, and psychoanalysis together in this particular realm of human experience, I have tried to shed

---

66. See in this connection the work of Garcia and Rodriguez (1989) regarding Argentinian and Salvadorian refugees, Cook and Timberlake (1989) regarding Vietnamese refugees, Mollica (1989) regarding other Indo-Chinese refugees, and the work of Dutch colleagues (Groenenberg 1999, Santini 1999, van Essen 1999, and van Waning 1999) regarding middle-Eastern refugees.

light on the experiential world of all immigrants, whether or not they figure in the clinical situation. I do not know how far I have succeeded in my effort, but I certainly have tried. The rest is now up to you, my readers. In the words of the renowned Urdu poet Jan Nisar Akhtar:

> Ab tum Jaano, ab tum samjho, chahey jaisa rung bharo
> Hum ne to ik naqsha Khencha, ik Khaka tayyar Kiya.
>
> [Now it is up to you; do what you wish, what you can.
> I have though prepared a sketch, a road map for you.]

In light of the fact that my book is about issues of temporo-spatial discontinuity, is it not interesting that I began this book by dedicating it to my U.S.-born children and am ending it by quoting a couplet by a man buried in Bombay, a man who was my beloved father?

GLOSSARY

A

Abhimanyu complex: Akhtar's designation for an individual's ability to migrate from his country and yet remain unable to return; named after a character in the famous Hindu epic *Mahabharata* who, while in utero, had heard his father reveal the secrets of entering a war to his mother but could not hear the tactics pertaining to exiting from the situation since his mother fell asleep.

Accidental immigrants: a term used by Elovitz and Kahn (1997) to describe individuals who arrive in a country for a visit but because of changed situations in the country of origin can no longer go back there.

Acculturation: the gradual process of autoplastic adaptation to post-migration changes in a variety of realms (e.g., topographical, biological, political, historical, economic, social, and psychological).

Acculturation gap: Prathikanti's (1997) term for the difference between older and younger members of an immigrant family in their familiarity and comfort with the culture of the country of adoption.

Adaptation: the capacity to cope appropriately and advantageously with one's environment. When the individual alters the environment to meet his needs, the resulting adaptation is called *alloplastic*. When, however, the individual modifies himself in response to the environment, the adaptation is called *autoplastic*.

Alienated identity: a term commonly used in the immigration literature for those who feel like misfits in both the ethnic community and the culture at large; generally applied to the adolescent offspring of immigrant parents, the term can also be applied to immigrants returning to their country of origin and finding themselves changed and unable to adjust there.

Alienation: a sense of estrangement from the emotional connections and values of one's family and society.

Amae: Japanese term that refers to an intermittent and culturally sanctioned interaction in which the customary rules of propriety are temporarily suspended, allowing people to seek, receive, and give affectionate support and indulgence to one another. "In shared enactments that are comparable to childhood creative make-believe play, the experiences of *amae* recall and transiently symbolically recreate the reassuring intimacy of the mother–child relationship of early childhood and the experiences of reunion and refueling of separation-individuation" (Freeman 1998, p. 47).

Amerocentric identity: Mehta's (1998) term for South Asian adolescents who grow up with strong North American values and are indifferent to their ethnic legacies; as adults, they are more likely to have intercultural marriages.

Anomie: a term coined by the renowned French sociologist Emile Durkheim (1858–1917) to describe the personal unrest and alienation that results from a major alteration or breakdown of social values and standards.

Assimilation: the process of losing ethnic rough edges and internalizing the cultural characteristics of the dominant group.

B

Bicultural punctuality: a term used by an unnamed University of Michigan graduate student for the immigrant's split allegiance to two psychosocial orientations toward time.

Bicultural self: a widely used expression in the immigration literature for the psychological self of immigrants (and their offspring), meant to denote the coexistence of behavioral attitudes and value systems emanating from two separate cultures; interestingly, some authors (e.g., Meaders 1997) use this term for a phase when the inner synthesis of two cultures is incomplete and conflictual, while others (e.g., Mehta 1998) use it to denote a state of relative harmony between the internalized dictates of the immigrant's two cultures.

Biculturalism: an ideology that puts a premium on including aspects of two separate cultures in consideration of life issues.

C

Collectivism: a politico-economic viewpoint advocating community control over production and distribution of goods.

Compromised identity: Mehta's (1998) term for what has been described above as "alienated identity"; a problematic outcome of adolescence characterized by a subjective sense of not belonging to either the culture of one's own ethnic group or that of the society at large.

Confederacy of selves: a term coined by Akhtar for an organization of self where culturally contradictory self-representations exist in a rather sequestered form.

Counterphobic assimilation: a term coined by Teja and Akhtar (1981) for an immigrant's tendency to rapidly renounce his original culture and adopt the characteristics of the new culture in order to avoid feeling different and therefore hurt and angry.

Cultural holding environment: Parens's (1998) extension of Winnicott's concept of the "holding environment," to include the silent but important role of social customs and rituals in ego development.

Cultural identity: the aspect of the core self-representation that is aligned and affiliated with the norms, attitudes, values, and communicative idioms of a group of people; while cultural identity is partly determined by ethnicity and religion, regional and linguistic variables perhaps play a larger role in its genesis. For instance, a Muslim from Bangladesh has a Bengali identity while a Muslim from Iraq has an Arab identity.

Culture: the customary and shared beliefs, attitudes, values, rituals, social forms, and practices of a religious, ethnic, racial, or regional group of people.

Culture shock: a term commonly used to describe the ego disturbance caused by a sudden and drastic change in the "average expectable environment" (Hartmann 1939); it puts the newcomer's personality to the test and challenges the stability of his psychic organization.

Culture-wise: Mehta's (1998) extension of the colloquialism "streetwise"; it refers to certain immigrant youngsters' capacity to skillfully utilize different behaviors in different cultural settings.

D

Deportee: one who has been removed or banished from a country by the order of its regime.

Desymbolizing effect: Grubrich-Simitis's (1984) concept pertaining to the impairment in the capacity to use and understand metaphors and higher connotative levels of language as a result of the distorted reality in political imprisonment and concentration camps.

Diaspora: the breaking up and scattering of a people.

Disenchantment of the promised land: an expression used by Grinberg and Grinberg (1989) for the occasionally intense feelings of disappointment felt by a recent immigrant in a new country.

Disorienting anxieties: a phrase coined by Grinberg and Grinberg (1989) to designate the inner and outer troubles resulting from a recent immigrant's failure to distinguish between the old and the new in the realm of his psychosocial existence.

Double mourning: a term used by van Essen (1999) to denote the dual task of an adolescent immigrant facing the loss of his country of origin, and, due to the developmentally appropriate pressures of individuation, the loss of internal support of his parents.

Dreams of transition: a phrase used by Meaders (1997) for manifest dreams that depict the acculturation process.

E

Emigration: leaving one's place of residence or country to live elsewhere.

Emigration without leaving home: a term coined by Kahn (1997c) for the situation in which a native begins to feel like a foreigner within his own country due to drastic and hostile political changes all around him.

Ethnicity: refers to the culture of a people and includes values, child-rearing practices, sense of history, modes of expression, and patterns of interpersonal behavior.

Ethnic identity: a feeling of belonging to a historical community; according to Thomson and colleagues (1993), ethnic identity is both positive ("we do this") and negative ("we do not do what they do"). It results from the exposure of a child to the family's cultural modes and its particular ways of conducting day-to-day life; identification with parents, especially during the oedipal phase, also enhances a sense of generational continuity, which is the cornerstone of later ethnic identity.

Ethnocentric identity: a term commonly found in the immigration literature that refers to the post-adolescent ethnocentricity that results in a feeling of comfort in the homoethnic milieu combined with discomfort in the sexual and vocational competitiveness of the culture at large.

Ethnocentric withdrawal: the tendency of some immigrants to lead a cloistered life and associate mainly or solely with people of their own ethnicity.

Ethnocentrism: the belief that the culture and people of one's ethnic group are inherently superior to others.

Ethnocultural self-representation: a term introduced in the literature by Bonovitz (1998) to link up the potentially overlapping ethnic and cultural aspects of identity *and* to keep it anchored in a metapsychological perspective.

Exile: an individual who takes up residence in a foreign country and who cannot visit his country of origin.

Experiences of efficacy: these emanate from "the awareness of having an initiating and causal role in bringing about states of needed responsiveness from others" (Wolf 1994, p. 73).

Extramural refueling: Akhtar's term for seeking emotional sustenance and rejuvenation by phone contact with friends and relatives in the country of origin or by actually visiting the homeland.

F

Fake refugees: a term used by Westermeyer (1990) for individuals who exploit the opportunity to assume the role of a refugee to solve immediate economic or legal problems.

Familial self: a term used by Roland (1988) to denote a psychic structure common in Asian Indians; this type of self is enmeshed with others and primarily experiences itself in relation to them.

Four tracks of post-immigration identity change: Akhtar's (1995) delineation of four dimensions along which the identity change following immigration occurs; the dimensions along with their metaphoric journeys include (1) drive and affects (from love or hate to ambivalence), (2) interpersonal and psychic space (from near or far to optimal distance), (3) temporality (from yesterday or tomorrow to today), and (4) social affiliation (from yours or mine to ours).

G

Genocide: the deliberate and systematic destruction of a racial, religious, ethnic, or cultural group of people.

H

Homoethnic community: a group of immigrant people belonging to the individual's own ethnic origin; by safeguarding traditions, celebrating festivals, building and maintaining places for religious and social gatherings, a community helps the individual maintain continuity with his original culture.

Hybrid identity: an expression common in the immigration literature and meant to denote the relatively smooth and successful admixture of bicultural attributes in the character and lifestyle of an immigrant.

Hyphenated identity: an expression frequently used to denote the immigrant's sense of himself as belonging partly to one culture and partly to another; it results in mixed and, at times, contradictory behaviors and attitudes.

I

Illegal aliens: immigrants who either have entered or have extended their stay in a foreign country without proper documents to permit them such privilege.

Immersion phase: Meaders's (1997) term for the early post-immigration period when feelings of loss are acute, anxiety is intense, and the struggle between regressive impulses and developmentally progressive demands is paramount.

Immigrant: one who has taken up residence in a region or country other than his place of birth.

Immigration: entering a region or country of which one is not a born native for purpose of residence.

Individualism: a doctrine asserting that all values, rights, and duties originate within an individual *and* that the interests of an individual are or ought to be ethically paramount.

Inner migration: has the same meaning as "emigration without leaving home" (see above).

Interior migration: a change of residence from one region to another culturally distinct region within the same country.

Intimacy gap: Roland's (1997) term for the difference that Indian immigrants feel exists between the depth of their friendships with fellow Indians and the depth of their friendships with fellow North Americans.

Intramural refueling: Akhtar's designation for the emotional sustenance immigrants draw from their contact with a homoethnic community.

Invisible immigrants: individuals who, because of skin color and linguistic similarity, are not generally recognized as different from the natives (Stephen Shanfield, personal communication); also used to describe those who deny their immigrant status because of intense guilt (Shokeid 1988).

L

Law of suspicious cultural intensity: phrase coined by Akhtar to underscore the fact that intensely felt cultural concerns frequently are unconscious covers for deeper intrapsychic conflicts.

M

Migration: moving from one country, region, locality, or place to another.

Mohajir: an Urdu word for immigrant; the designation for those Muslims in Pakistan who migrated to the region at the time of British India's partition into India and Pakistan.

Money-hypochondria: a term introduced by Grinberg and Grinberg (1989) for the exaggerated fear of poverty seen in traumatized immigrants.

Mourning–liberation process: a term coined by Pollock (1989) for the Janus-faced nature of response to trauma: on the one hand it causes grief, and on the other it opens up new vistas of life experience by freeing the person from early objects.

Multiple splitting: Groenenberg's (1999) concept that describes the immigrant's resorting to "all good" and "all bad" views of his country of adoption and country of origin *in addition to* splitting the image of his country of origin itself into "all good" and "all bad" versions.

Multisensory bridges: a concept developed by Brenner (1988) to describe a response to traumatic loss in which early developmentally appropriate sensory experiences are revived in memory and used to re-create the illusion of being with lost loved ones; while originally introduced in the context of children who survived the Holocaust and who were traumatically separated from their parents, the concept can indeed be extended to explain certain psychosomatic features of the experience of nostalgia in general.

N

Negative acculturation: the propensity of alienated and anguished immigrant and first-generation youth to selectively identify with the most starkly undesirable aspects (e.g., drugs, guns, violence) of their adopted culture.

Negative nostalgia: the preoccupation of some exiles and refugees with how *bad* their country of origin was.

Nostalgia: an excessively sentimental yearning for times and places left behind; colloquially referred to as "homesickness."

O

Oleh: one who rises in esteem by migrating to Israel.

P

Perceptual bath: a term coined by Awad (unpublished discussion of Akhtar's [1995a] paper, October 1995) for the holding function of smells, sounds, and visual texture of the early environment; its relatively silent internalization provides a background screen for all subsequent perceptions.

Phasic assimilation: the immigrant's tendency to oscillate between ethnic and assimilated lifestyles over a long span of time.

Poisoning of nostalgia: a term coined by Akhtar for the retrograde spread of aggression causing a blocked access to prior good memories; common in situations of grossly traumatic departures.

Polyglottism: acquisition of a second language during adulthood.

Polylingualism: acquisition of more than one language from early childhood onward.

Pragmatic assimilation: a superficial adjustment to the new culture with little psychological internalization; the social and the psychic selves thus come to live separate and dissociative lives.

Prejudice: an adverse opinion, leaning, or attitude formed without just grounds and before accumulating sufficient knowledge pertinent to the context.

Protective rite of farewell: phrase used by Grinberg and Grinberg (1989) to underscore the fact that the opportunity to say "goodbye" to loved people and places lessens the trauma of leaving.

Proxy-base for refueling: term coined by Akthar (1995) for a place or country that can stand for the lost home and therefore provide emotional sustenance to those who have lost their original sources for refueling.

R

Racism: a belief that race is the fundamental determinant of human traits and abilities and that racial differences imply an inherent superiority of one group of human beings over another.

Refugee: an individual who has sought shelter in a foreign country to escape natural danger or ethnopolitical persecution in the country of origin.

Return to fire: a phrase used by Brenner (1999) to denote the visiting of Nazi concentration camps by their survivors.

S

Satellite state: Volkan and Corney's (1968) term for the psychological state in which an individual fears both progression and regression in the realm of autonomy and exists as a captive body orbiting within the gravitational field of an intense, though ambivalent, dependency.

Sensory denial: term used by Knafo and Yaari (1997) for the continuation, after emigration, of a perceptual sense that one is still living in one's country of origin.

Sedentary migration: term used by Grinberg and Grinberg (1989) for the deliberate move after immigration to a carefully chosen place that resembles one's country of origin in its topography and climate.

Shared ethnic scotoma: Shapiro and Pinsker's (1973) phrase for blind spots in the therapeutic alliance and countertransference collusions with the patient when the therapist and the patient are of the same ethnicity; under such circumstances deeper understanding of the patient's psychopathology can suffer and aggression can be displaced onto ethnoculturally different others.

Social denial: a term used by Knafo and Yaari (1997) for the situation where one continues to speak in one's original language and to associate with fellow immigrants from one's country of origin in anxious refusal to deal with changed realities.

Structural violence: term coined by Schreuder (1999) to denote the psychostructurally deleterious effect of political confinement and torture; such violence breaks through the boundaries of the self and the source of the destructive stimulus can then just as easily be ascribed to the self as to the external object causing it.

T

Teacher transference: Taketomo's (1989) designation of the Japanese analysand's respectful desires to be mentored by his or her analyst; the basis of such feelings is in the important connection a Japanese child makes with the kindergarten teacher (often a male!) since he is the first major extra-familial and truly paternal object in the child's experience. A subtle implication here is that Japanese fathers are often more maternal and hence the child's first "father-like" experience occurs in the relationship with the kindergarten teacher.

Temporal fracture of the self: an experiential discontinuity between the memories, feelings, and relationships one had in different eras of one's life.

Third individuation: Akhtar's (1995a) term for the reformulation of identity after the mourning–liberation process of immigration; an extrapolation of Mahler's (1958b) concept of separation-individuation in childhood and Blos's (1967) term, the "second-individuation process" of adolescence.

Third reality: a term used by Mehta (1998) to refer to the immigrant youth's psychosocial space which, culturally speaking, is "neither of his or her parents' homeland nor of the adopted land, but uniquely and historically different" (p. 137).

Time binding: Beiser's (1980) term for the ego's attempts to maintain connectedness and links between the past, present, and future; this is disrupted in immigrants and refugees; time is often experienced by them as stagnating or fragmented.

Time collapse: Volkan's (1997) term for the rupture of boundaries between the past and present; the emotions and perceptions associated with the past begin to be experienced as if the trauma has just occurred and they are even projected onto the future. What is remembered, felt, and expected come together.

Time dominance: Beiser's (1980) term for the predominant valence of a particular era (past, present, or future) in an individual's psychic life; in immigrants and refugees, the past continues to dominate the present and there is little affective investment in the future.

Time of the heart: an expression coined by Akhtar to underscore that in non-Western cultures, the predominant concern for loved ones is the crucial factor determining the timings of social events; also known as "time of love."

Time of the mind: an expression coined by Akhtar to highlight that, in industrialized societies, the concern for efficiency and productivity is the crucial factor in setting the time of social events; also known as "time of money."

Transcultural identity: a term reserved by Nobuko Meaders for the third and final phase (the earlier two being "survival of identity" and "bicultural identity") of the impact of immigration upon identity; in this phase, bicultural attitudes no longer feel conflictual and the individual feels a sense of belonging to both of his cultures.

Transitional actions: a term used by Groenenberg (1999) for individual and collective behaviors of immigrants and refugees (e.g., political gatherings, music, cultural festivals) intended to bridge the gap between their countries of origin and of adoption.

U

U.S. Immigration Act of 1965: this act rendered obsolete the quota system based upon nationalities of origin for granting residence in the United States.

U.S. Immigration Act of 1990: this act formally removed homosexuality as a basis for exclusion in granting residence in the United States.

W

We-self: a term used by Roland (1996) to denote the intrapsychic experience of Asian Indians whereby the persons live in an on-going state of partial merger with others, with an emotional flow back and forth.

Wound of return: expression coined by the Spanish journalist Maruja Torres (cited by Grinberg and Grinberg 1989) to denote the disappointments and difficulties faced by the immigrant who moves back to his original country; the person himself is changed and the country is no longer what he left behind, making the "return" yet another immigration.

X

Xenophobia: fear and avoidance of strangers and anything that seems foreign and alien to one's experience.

Y

Yored: the somewhat derogatory Hebrew term for those emigrating from Israel to other countries.

Z

Zionism: an international sociopolitical movement originated for the establishment of a Jewish national or religious community in Palestine and later for the support of modern Israel.

REFERENCES

Aarif, I. (1983). *Meher-e-doneem*, p. 87. Karachi, Pakistan: Maktaba Danyal.

Abbasi, A. (1997). *When two worlds collide in the psychoanalytic space.* Paper presented at the American Psychoanalytic Association Fall Meetings, New York, NY, December.

———— (1998). Speaking the unspeakable. In *Blacks and Jews on the Couch: Psychoanalytic Reflections on Black–Jewish Conflict,* ed. A. Helmreich and P. Marcus, pp. 133–147. Westport, CT: Praeger.

Abelin, E. L. (1971). The role of the father in the separation-individuation process. In *Separation-Individuation: Essays in Honor of Margaret Mahler,* ed. J. B. McDevitt and C. F. Settlage, pp. 229–253. New York: International Universities Press.

Abraham, K. (1911). On the determining power of names. In *Clinical Papers and Essays on Psychoanalysis,* pp. 31–32. New York: Brunner/Mazel.

Abse, D. W. (1966). *Hysteria and Related Mental Disorders.* Bristol: John Wright and Sons.

Adler, G. (1985). *Borderline Psychopathology and Its Treatment.* New York: Jason Aronson.

Ahmad, I. (1997). Geriatric psychopathology. In *A Guide to Clinical Assessment,* ed. W. Tseng and J. Strelver, pp. 223–240. New York: Brunner/Mazel.

Akhtar S. (1984). The syndrome of identity diffusion. *American Journal of Psychiatry* 141:1381–1385.

———— (1988) Four culture-bound psychiatric syndromes in India. *International Journal of Social Psychiatry* 34:70–74.

———— (1991). Three fantasies related to unresolved separation-individuation: a less recognized aspect of severe character pathology. In *Beyond the Symbiotic Orbit: Advances in Separation-Individuation Theory—Essays in Honor of Selma Kramer, M.D.*, ed. S. Akhtar and H. Parens, pp. 261–284. Hillsdale, NJ: Analytic Press.

———— (1992a). Tethers, orbits and invisible fences: clinical, developmental, sociocultural, and technical aspects of optimal distance. In *When the Body Speaks: Psychological Meanings in Kinetic Clues*, ed. S. Kramer and S. Akhtar, pp. 21–57. Northvale, NJ: Jason Aronson.

———— (1992b). *Broken Structures: Severe Personality Disorders and Their Treatment.* Northvale, NJ: Jason Aronson.

———— (1994). Object constancy and adult psychopathology. *International Journal of Psycho-Analysis* 75:441–455.

———— (1995a). A third individuation: immigration, identity, and the psychoanalytic process. *Journal of the American Psychoanalytic Association* 43:1051–1084.

———— (1995b). *Quest for Answers: A Primer for Understanding and Treating Severe Personality Disorders.* Northvale, NJ: Jason Aronson.

———— (1996). "Someday . . ." and "if only . . ." fantasies: pathological optimism and inordinate nostalgia as related forms of idealization. *Journal of the American Psychoanalytic Association* 44:723–753.

———— (1997). Review of *All the Mothers are One: Hindu India and the Cultural Reshaping of Psychoanalysis*, by Stanley Kurtz. *Journal of the American Psychoanalytic Association* 45:1014–1019.

———— (1998a). From simplicity through contradiction to paradox: the evolving psychic reality of the borderline patient in treatment. *International Journal of Psycho-Analysis* 79:241–252.

———— (1998b). Psychoanalysis and the rainbow of cultural authenticity. In *The Colors of Childhood: Separation-Individuation Across Cultural, Racial, and Ethnic Differences*, pp. 113–128. Northvale, NJ: Jason Aronson.

———— (1999a). Review of *Immigrant Experiences: Personal Narrative and Psychological Analysis*, edited by P. Elovitz and C. Kahn. In *Mind and Human Interaction* 10:57–60.

———— (1999b). The immigrant, the exile and the experience of nostalgia. *Journal of Applied Psychoanalytic Studies* 1(2):123–130.

———— (1999c). Transformation of identity upon immigration: recapitulation and reconsideration. In *Proceedings of the IPA–UNESCO Congress: At the Threshold of the Millennium*, Lima, Peru, April 1998 (in press).

———— (1999d). *Inner Torment: Living Between Conflict and Fragmentation*. Northvale, NJ: Jason Aronson.

———— (1999e). Age at migration: an introductory overview. *Mind and Human Interaction* 10:3–10.

Akhtar, S., and Brown, J. (1999). Animals in psychiatric symptomatology. In *Mental Zoo: Animals in the Human Mind and Its Pathology*, ed. S. Akhtar and V. D. Volkan. Madison, CT: International Universities Press.

Akhtar, S., and Byrne, J. P. (1983). The concept of splitting and its clinical relevance. *American Journal of Psychiatry* 140:1016–1018.

Akhtar, S., and Kramer, S. (1999). Beyond the parental orbit: brothers, sisters, and others. In *Brothers and Sisters: Developmental, Dynamic and Technical Aspects of the Sibling Relationship*, ed. S. Akhtar and S. Kramer, pp. 1–24. Northvale, NJ: Jason Aronson.

Akhtar, S., and Samuel, S. (1996). The concept of identity: developmental origins, phenomenology, clinical relevance, and measurement. *Harvard Review of Psychiatry* 3:254–267.

Akhtar, S., and Smolar, A. (1998). Visiting the father's grave. *Psychoanalytic Quarterly* 67:474–483.

Akhtar, S., and Volkan, V. D., eds. (1999a). *Mental Zoo: Animals in the Human Mind and Its Pathology*. Madison, CT: International Universities Press.

———— (1999b). *Cultural Zoo: Animals in the Human Mind and Its Sublimations*. Madison, CT: Psychosocial Press.

Altman, L. L. (1977). Some vicissitudes of love. *Journal of the American Psychoanalytic Association* 95:35–52.

Amati-Mehler, J., Argentieri, S., and Canestri, J. (1993). *The Babel of the Unconscious: Mother Tongue and Foreign Languages in the Psychoanalytic Dimension*, trans. J. Whitelaw-Cucco. Madison, CT: International Universities Press.

Amirthanayagam, I. (1995). What happened to all my life. In *Living in America: Poetry and Fiction by South Asian American Writers*, ed. R. Rustomji-Kerns, pp. 37–38. Boulder, CO: Westview.

Antokolitz, J. C. (1993). A psychoanalytic view of cross-cultural passages. *American Journal of Psychoanalysis* 53:35–54.

Anzieu, D. (1976). Narciso, la envoltora sonora bel si mismo. *Nouvelle Revue de Psychoanalyse* 13.

Apprey, M. (1993). The African-American experience: forced immigration and the transgenerational trauma. *Mind and Human Interaction* 4:70–75.

———— (1999). Reinventing the self in the face of received transgenerational hatred in the African-American community. *Journal of Applied Psychoanalytic Studies* 1:131–143.

Awad, G. (1995). Discussion of "A Third Individuation: Immigration, Identity, and the Psychoanalytic Process," by S. Akhtar, Michigan Psychoanalytic Society, Detroit, MI, October 7 (unpublished).

Babcock, C., and Caudill, W. (1958). Personal and cultural factors in treating a Nisei man. In *Clinical Studies in Culture Conflict*, ed. G. Seward. New York: Ronald.

Bach, S. (1985). *Narcissistic States and the Therapeutic Process*. New York: Jason Aronson.

Bachrach, H., and Leaff, L. (1978). "Analyzability": a systematic review of the clinical and quantitative literature. *Journal of the American Psychoanalytic Association* 26:881–920.

Bakhtin, M. M. (1986). *Speech Genres and Other Late Essays*, trans. V. W. McGee. Austin, TX: University of Texas Press.

———— (1990). *Art and Answerability*, trans. V. Liapunov. Austin, TX: University of Texas Press.

Balint, M. (1959). *Thrills and Regressions*. London: Hogarth.

———— (1968). *The Basic Fault*. London: Tavistock.

Batchelor, I. R. C. (1969). *Henderson and Gillespie's Textbook of Psychiatry*, 10th ed. London: Oxford University Press.

Baxter, J. K. (1958). *In Fires of No Return*. London: Oxford University Press.

Beiser, M. (1980). Coping with past and future: a study of adaptation to social change in West Africa. *Journal of Operational Psychiatry* 11:140–154.

———— (1990). Mental health of refugees in resettlement countries. In *Mental Health of Immigrants and Refugees*, ed. W. H. Holtzman and T. H. Bornemann, pp. 51–65. Austin TX: University of Texas Press.

Beiser, M., and Hyman, I. (1997). Refugees' time perspective and mental health. *American Journal of Psychiatry* 154:996–1002.

Benedek, T. (1970). Fatherhood and parenthood. In *Parenthood: Its Psychology and Psychopathology*, ed. E. J. Anthony and T. Benedek, pp. 169–183. Boston, MA: Little, Brown.

Bennani, J., ed. (1985). *Du Bilinguisme*. Paris: Denoel.

Bergman, A. (1980). Ours, yours, mine. In *Rapprochement: The Critical Subphase of Separation-Individuation*, ed. R. F. Lax, S. Bach, and J. A. Burland, pp. 199–216. New York: Jason Aronson.

Berry, J. W. (1990). Acculturation and adaptation: a general framework. In *Mental Health of Immigrants and Refugees*, ed. W. H. Holtzman and T. H. Bornemann, pp. 90–102. Austin TX: University of Texas Press.

Bick, E. (1968). The experience of the skin in early object relations. *International Journal of Psycho-Analysis* 49:484–486.

Bion, W. (1967). *Second Thoughts*. New York: Jason Aronson.

Bleuler, E. (1908). *Textbook of Psychiatry*, trans. A. A. Brill. New York: Macmillan.

Blos, P. (1962). *On Adolescence*. New York: Free Press.

——— (1965). The initial stage of male adolescence. *Psychoanalytic Study of the Child* 20:145–164. New York: International Universities Press.

——— (1967). The second individuation process of adolescence. *Psychoanalytic Study of the Child* 22:162–186. New York: International Universities Press.

——— (1974). The genealogy of the ego ideal. *Psychoanalytic Study of the Child* 29:43–88. New Haven, CT: Yale University Press.

——— (1984). Father and son. *Journal of the American Psychoanalytic Association* 32:301–324.

——— (1985). *Son and Father: Before and Beyond the Oedipus Complex*. New York: Free Press.

Blum, H. P. (1977). The prototype of preoedipal reconstruction. *Journal of the American Psychoanalytic Association* 25:757–785.

——— (1981). Object constancy and paranoid conspiracy. *Journal of the American Psychoanalytic Association* 29:789–813.

——— (1985). Superego formation, adolescent transformation, and the adult neurosis. *Journal of the American Psychoanalytic Association* 33:887–909.

Bonovitz, J. (1998). Reflections of the self in the cultural looking glass. In *The Colors of Childhood: Separation-Individuation Across Cultural, Racial, and Ethnic Differences*, ed. S. Akhtar and S. Kramer, pp. 169–198. Northvale, NJ: Jason Aronson.

Bonovitz, J., and Ergas, R. (1999). The affective experience of the child immigrant: issues of loss and mourning. *Mind and Human Interaction* 10:15–25.

Bouvet, M. (1958). Technical variations and the concept of distance. *International Journal of Psycho-Analysis* 39:211–221.

Bowlby, J. (1969). *Attachment and Loss: Vol. I: Attachment*. London: Hogarth.

Boyer B., and Giovacchini P. L. (1980). *Psychoanalytic Treatment of Characterological and Schizophrenic Disorders*. New York: Jason Aronson.

Brenner, C. (1979). Working alliance, therapeutic alliance and transference. *Journal of the American Psychoanalytic Association* 27:137–157.

Brenner, I. (1988). Multi-sensory bridges in response to object loss. *Psycho-analytic Review* 75:573–587.

———— (1999). Returning to the fire: surviving the Holocaust and "going back." *Journal of Applied Psychoanalytic Studies* 1(2):145–162.

Breuer J., and Freud S. (1893–1895). *Studies on Hysteria,* trans. J. Strachey. New York: Basic Books, 1957.

Brodsky, J. (1973). Elegy: for Robert Lowell. In *A Part of Speech,* pp. 135–137. New York: Farrar, Straus and Giroux.

Brody, E. B. (1973). *The Lost Ones: Social Forces and Mental Illness in Rio de Janeiro.* New York: International Universities Press.

Burland, A. (1986). Illusion, reality, and fantasy. In *Self and Object Constancy,* ed. R. F. Lax, S. Bach, and J. A. Burland, pp. 291–303. New York: Guilford.

Buxbaum, E. (1949). The role of a second language in the formation of ego and superego. *Psychoanalytic Quarterly* 18:279–289.

Cafavy, C. P. (1906). Returning from Greece. In *C. P. Cafavy: Collected Poems,* ed. G. Savidis, trans. E. Keeley and P. Sherrard, p. 369. Princeton, NJ: Princeton University Press.

Cain, A. C., and Cain, B. S. (1964). On replacing a child. *Journal of the American Academy of Child Psychiatry* 3:443–456.

Carlin, J. (1990). Refugee and immigrant populations at special risk. In *Mental Health of Immigrants and Refugees,* ed. W. H. Holtzman and T. H. Bornemann, pp. 224–233. Austin TX: University of Texas Press.

Casement, P. J. (1982). Samuel Beckett's relationship to his mother-tongue. *International Review of Psycho-Analysis* 9:35–44.

———— (1991). *Learning from the Patient.* New York: Guilford.

Cath, S. (1997). Loss and restitution in late life. In *The Seasons of Life: Separation-Individuation Perspectives,* ed. S. Akhtar and S. Kramer, pp. 127–156. Northvale, NJ: Jason Aronson.

Cavenar, J. O., and Nash. J. L. (1976). The dream as a signal for termination. *Journal of the American Psychoanalytic Association* 24:425–436.

Chasseguet-Smirgel, J. (1984). *Creativity and Perversion.* New York: Norton.

———— (1985). *The Ego Ideal: A Psychoanalytic Essay on the Malady of the Ideal.* New York: Norton.

Cheng, F. (1985). Le cas du chinois. In *Du Bilinguisme,* ed. J. Bennani. Paris: Denoel.

Cioran, E. M. (1982). *Storia e Utopia.* Milan: Adelphi.

Colarusso, C. A. (1990). The third individuation: the effect of biological parenthood on separation-individuation processes in adulthood.

Psychoanalytic Study of the Child 45:179–194. New Haven, CT: Yale University Press.

———— (1997). Separation-individuation processes in middle adulthood: the fourth individuation. In *The Seasons of Life: Separation-Individuation Perspectives*, ed. S. Akhtar and S. Kramer, pp. 73–94. Northvale, NJ: Jason Aronson.

Coles, R. (1967). *The South Goes North: Volume III of Children of Crisis.* Boston, MA: Little, Brown.

Cook, K. O., and Timberlake, E. M. (1989). Cross-cultural counseling with Vietnamese refugees. In *Crossing Cultures in Mental Health*, ed. D. R. Koslow and E. P. Salett, pp. 84–100. Washington, DC: SIETAR International.

Cooper, D. (1995). I have been offered my country's begging bowl again. In *Living in America: Poetry and Fiction by South Asian American Writers*, ed. R. Rustomji-Kerns, pp. 41–42. Boulder, CO: Westview.

Copelman, D. (1993). The immigrant experience: margin notes. *Mind and Human Interaction* 4:76–82.

Crusz, R. (1995). Conversations with God about my present whereabouts. In *Living in America: Poetry and Fiction by South Asian American Writers*, ed. R. Rustomji-Kerns, pp. 43–45. Boulder, CO: Westview.

Denford, S. (1981). Going away. *International Journal of Psycho-Analysis* 59:325–332.

Deutsch, H. (1942). Some forms of emotional disturbance and their relationship to schizophrenia. *Psychoanalytic Quarterly* 11:301–321.

DeVos, G. (1980). Afterword. In *The Quiet Therapies*, D. K. Reynolds, pp. 113–132. Honolulu: University of Hawaii Press.

Diagnostic and Statistical Manual for Mental Disorders (1994), 4th ed. Washington, DC: American Psychiatric Association.

Diaz-Perez, R. (1986). Memories. In *Anthology of Contemporary Latin American Literature 1960–1984*, ed. B. J. Luby and W. H. Finke, p. 126. Cranbury, NJ: Associated University Presses.

Diefendorf, A. R. (1921). *Clinical Psychiatry.* London: Macmillan.

Doi, T. (1973). *The Anatomy of Dependence.* Tokyo: Kodansha International.

Dunn, J. (1995). Intersubjectivity in psychoanalysis: a critical review. *International Journal of Psycho-Analysis* 76:723–738.

Edwards, J., Ruskin, N., and Turrini, P. (1981). *Separation-Individuation Theory and Application.* New York: Gardner.

Eisnitz, A. (1980). The organization of the self representation and its influence on pathology. *Psychoanalytic Quarterly* 49:361–392.

Elovitz, P. H., and Kahn, C. (1997). *Immigrant Experiences: Personal Narrative and Psychological Analysis.* Cranbury, NJ: Associated University Presses.

Emde, R. N. (1983). The prerepresentational self and its affective core. *Psychoanalytic Study of the Child* 38:165–192. New Haven, CT: Yale University Press.

Erikson, E. H. (1950a). Growth and crises of the healthy personality. In *Identity and the Life Cycle,* pp. 50–100. New York: International Universities Press, 1959.

——— (1950b). *Childhood and Society.* New York: Norton.

——— (1954). The dream specimen of psychoanalysis. *Journal of the American Psychoanalytic Association* 2:5–56.

——— (1956). The problem of ego identity. In *Identity and the Life Cycle,* pp. 104–164. New York: International Universities Press, 1959.

——— (1958). *Young Man Luther: A Study in Psychoanalysis and History.* New York: Norton.

——— (1959). *Childhood and Society.* Boston: Little Brown.

——— (1962). *Identity: Youth and Crisis.* New York: Norton.

Escoll, P. J. (1977). Panel report: the contribution of psychoanalytic developmental concepts to adult analysis. *Journal of the American Psychoanalytic Association* 25:219–234.

——— (1992). Vicissitudes of optimal distance through the life cycle. In *When the Body Speaks: Psychological Meanings in Kinetic Clues,* ed. S. Kramer and S. Akhtar, pp. 59–87. Northvale, NJ: Jason Aronson.

Ewing, C. (1991). Can psychoanalytic theories explain the Pakistani woman? Intrapsychic autonomy and interpersonal engagement in the extended family. *Ethos* 19:131–160.

Fairbairn, W. R. D. (1952). *Psychoanalytic Studies of the Personality.* London: Tavistock.

Falk, A. (1974). Border symbolism. *Psychoanalytic Quarterly* 43:650–660.

Fenichel, O. (1945). *The Psychoanalytic Theory of Neurosis.* New York: Norton.

Ferenczi, S. (1911). On obscene words. In *Final Contributions to the Problems and Methods of Psycho-Analysis.* London: Hogarth.

Filet, B. (1998). Psychoanalysis after Babel: the communication between psychoanalysts of different cultures and its problems. *Psychoanalysis in Europe* 51:36–53.

Fischer, N. (1971). An interracial analysis: transference and countertransference significance. *Journal of the American Psychoanalytic Association* 19:736–745.

Fischer, N., and Fischer, R. M. S. (1991). Adolescence, sex, and neurosogenesis: a clinical perspective. In *Beyond the Symbiotic Orbit: Advances in Separation-Individuation Theory—Essays in Honor of Selma Kramer, M.D.*, ed. S. Akhtar and H. Parens, pp. 209–226. Hillsdale, NJ: Analytic Press.

Fish, F. J. (1964). *An Outline of Psychiatry.* Bristol: John Wright and Sons.

Flegenheimer, F. (1989). Languages and psychoanalysis: the polyglot patient and the polyglot analyst. *International Review of Psycho-Analysis* 16:377–383.

Fleming, J. (1972). Early object deprivation and transference phenomena: the working alliance. *Psychoanalytic Quarterly* 21: 23–49.

Fodor, N. (1950). Varieties of nostalgia. *Psychoanalytic Review* 37:25–38.

Fonagy, P., and Target, M. (1997). Attachment and reflective function: their role in self-organization. *Development and Psychopathology* 9:679–700.

Frankl, V. (1959). *Man's Search for Meaning.* New York: Washington Square Press.

Freedman, A. (1956). The feeling of nostalgia and its relationship to phobia. *Bulletin of the Philadelphia Association for Psychoanalysis* 6:84–92.

Freeman, D. (1997). *Precocity, separation-individuation, refueling, and amae.* Paper presented at the American Psychoanalytic Associations' Interdisciplinary Conference, *Amae* Reconsidered, San Diego, CA, May 18.

——— (1998). Emotional refueling in development, mythology, and cosmology: the Japanese separation-individuation experience. In *The Colors of Childhood: Separation-Individuation Across Cultural, Racial, and Ethnic Differences*, ed. S. Akhtar and S. Kramer, pp. 17–60. Northvale, NJ: Jason Aronson.

——— (in press). Cross-cultural perspectives on the bond between man and animals. In *Cultural Zoo: Animals in the Human Mind and Its Sublimations.* Madison, CT: Psychosocial Press.

Freud, S. (1900). Interpretation of dreams. *Standard Edition* 4:1–337.

——— (1905). Jokes and their relation to the unconscious. *Standard Edition* 8:9–236.

——— (1908). On the sexual theories of children. *Standard Edition* 9:207–234.

——— (1909). Analysis of a phobia in a five year old boy. *Standard Edition* 10:5–149.

——— (1911). Formulations on the two principles of mental functioning. *Standard Edition* 12:218–230.

———— (1912). Recommendations to physicians practising psycho-analysis. *Standard Edition* 12:111–122.

———— (1917). Mourning and melancholia. *Standard Edition* 14:237–258.

———— (1920). Beyond the pleasure principle. *Standard Edition* 18:7–68.

———— (1921). Group psychology and the analysis of the ego. *Standard Edition* 18:67–144.

———— (1923). The ego and the id. *Standard Edition* 19:12–68.

———— (1924). The dissolution of the Oedipus compex. *Standard Edition* 19:173–179.

———— (1925). Some psychical consequences of the anatomical distinction between the sexes. *Standard Edition* 19:243–258.

———— (1926a). Address to the society of B'nai B'rith. *Standard Edition* 20:271–274.

———— (1926b). Inhibitions, symptoms and anxiety. *Standard Edition* 20:1–260.

———— (1927). The future of an illusion. *Standard Edition* 21:5–56.

———— (1930). Civilization and its discontents. *Standard Edition* 21:64–145.

———— (1933). New introductory lectures on psychoanalysis. *Standard Edition* 22:5–158.

Fromm, E. (1950). *Psychoanalysis and Religion.* New Haven, CT: Yale University Press.

Fu, L. (1956). Outside the window. In *Anthology of Modern Chinese Poetry,* ed. M. Yeh, p. 88. New Haven, CT: Yale University Press, 1992.

Gaddini, E. (1972). Aggression and the pleasure principle: towards a psychoanalytic theory of aggression. *International Journal of Psycho-Analysis* 53:191–197.

Galenson E., and Roiphe, H. (1971). The impact of early sexual discovery on mood, defensive organization, and symbolization. *Psychoanalytic Study of the Child* 26:195–216. New Haven, CT: Yale University Press.

Garcia, M. O., and Rodriguez, P. F. (1989). Psychological effects of political repression in Argentina and El Salvador. In *Crossing Cultures in Mental Health,* ed. D. R. Koslow and E. P. Salett, pp. 64–83. Washington, DC: SIETAR International.

Garza-Guerrero, A. C. (1974). Culture shock: its mourning and the vicissitudes of identity. *Journal of the American Psychoanalytic Association* 22:408–429.

Gay, P. (1988). *Freud: A Life for Our Time.* New York: Norton.

Ghalib, A. U. K. (1841). *Diwan-e-Ghalib.* New Delhi: Maktaba Jamia Ltd., 1969.

Goldberg, E., Myers, W. A., and Zeifman, I. (1974). Some observations on three interracial analyses. *International Journal of Psycho-Analysis* 55:495–500.

Gonzalez, F. J., and Espin, O. M. (1996). Latino men, Latina women, and homosexuality. In *Textbook of Homosexuality and Mental Health*, ed. R. P. Cabaj and T. S. Stein, pp. 583–602. Washington, DC: American Psychiatric Press.

Gorkin, M. (1996). Countertransference in cross-cultural psychotherapy. In *Reaching Across Boundaries of Culture and Class*, ed. R. Pérez Foster, M. Moskowitz, and R. A. Javier, pp. 47–70. Northvale, NJ: Jason Aronson.

Green, R. (1975). Sexual identity research strategies. *Archives of Sexual Behavior* 4:337–352.

Greenacre, P. (1957). The childhood of the artist. *Psychoanalytic Study of the Child* 12:47–65. New York: International Universities Press.

——— (1966). Problems of overidealization of the analyst and of analysis: their manifestations in the transference and countertransference relationship. *Psychoanalytic Study of the Child* 21:193–212. New York: International Universities Press.

——— (1975). On reconstruction. *Journal of the American Psychoanalytic Association* 23:693–712.

Greenson, R. R. (1950). The mother tongue and the mother. *International Journal of Psycho-Analysis* 31:18–23.

——— (1954). About the sound "mm . . ." *Psychoanalytic Quarterly* 22:234–239.

——— (1965). The working alliance and the transference neurosis. *Psychoanalytic Quarterly* 34:155–181.

——— (1968). Disidentifying from mother. *International Journal of Psycho-Analysis* 49:370–374.

Grinberg, L., and Grinberg, R. (1989). *Psychoanalytic Perspectives on Migration and Exile*, trans. N. Festinger. New Haven, CT: Yale University Press.

Grinker R., Werble B., and Drye R. C. (1968). *The Borderline Patient*. New York: Jason Aronson.

Groenenberg, M. (1999). Flight, acculturation, longing to return, and identity: struggles in the interpersonal and psychic space. *Proceedings of the IPA–UNESCO Congress: At the Threshold of the Millennium*, Lima, Peru, April 1998 (in press).

Grotstein, J. S. (1981). *Splitting and Projective Identification*. New York: Jason Aronson.

Grubrich-Simitis, I. (1984). From concretism to metaphor: thoughts on some theoretical and technical aspects of the psychoanalytic work with children of Holocaust survivors. *Psychoanalytic Study of the Child* 39: 301–319. New Haven, CT: Yale University Press.

Gunderson, J. G. (1985). *Borderline Personality Disorder*. Washington, DC: American Psychiatric Press.

Gunderson, J. G., and Singer, M. (1975). Defining borderline patients: an overview. *American Journal of Psychiatry* 133:1–10.

Guntrip, H. (1969). *Schizoid Phenomena, Object Relations and the Self*. New York: International Universities Press.

Guttman, S. A., Jones, R. L., and Parrish, S. M. (1980). *The Concordance to the Standard Edition of the Complete Psychological Works of Sigmund Freud*, vol I. Boston, MA: G. K. Hall.

Haley, A. (1976). *Roots*. New York: Doubleday.

Hall, E. (1973). *Silent Language*. New York: Doubleday.

Handlin, O. (1973). *The Uprooted: The Epic Story of the Great Migration That Made the American People*. Boston, MA: Little, Brown.

Harris, M. (1993). Performing the other's text: Bakhtin and the art of cross-cultural hermeneutics. *Mind and Human Interaction* 4:92–97.

Hartmann, H. (1939). *Ego Psychology and the Problem of Adaptation*, ed. D. Rapaport. New York: International Universities Press, 1958.

——— (1959). Comments on the psychoanalytic theory of the ego. In *Essays on Ego Psychology*, pp. 113–141. New York: International Universities Press.

——— (1964). *Essays on Ego Psychology*. New York: International Universities Press.

Hinsie, L. E., and Campbell, R. J. (1975). *Psychiatric Dictionary*, 4th Edition. New York: Oxford University Press.

Hoffman, E. (1989). *Lost in Translation: A Life in a New Language*. New York: Dutton.

Hoffman, I. Z. (1992). Some practical implications of a social constructivist view of the psychoanalytic situation. *Psychoanalytic Dialogues* 2:287–304.

Hojat, M., Shapurian, R., Nayerahmadi, H., et al. (1999). Premarital sexual, child rearing, and family attitudes of Iranian men and women in the United States and Iran. *The Journal of Psychology* 133:19–31.

Holmes, D. E. (1992). Race and transference in psychoanalysis and psychotherapy. *International Journal of Psycho-Analysis* 73:1–11.

——— (1994). Discussion of "A Third Individuation: Immigration, Identity, and the Psychoanalytic Process," by S. Akhtar, presented at the

14th Annual Division 39 Spring Meeting of the American Psychological Association, Washington, DC, April 13–17 (unpublished).

Horney, K. (1937). *The Neurotic Personality of Our Time*. New York: Norton.

Hovey, J. D., and King, C. A. (1996). Acculturative stress, depression, and suicidal ideation among immigrant and second generation Latino adolescents *Journal of the American Academy of Child and Adolescent Psychiatry* 35:1183–1192.

Howell, N. (1999). The poisoning of nostalgia: commentary. *Journal of Applied Psychoanalytic Studies* 1:163–168.

Hsu, F. L. K. (1953). *American and Chinese: Two Ways of Life*. New York: Henry Schuman.

Hughes, C. (1993). Culture in clinical psychiatry. In *Culture, Ethnicity and Mental Illness*, ed. A. C. Gaw, pp. 3–42. Washington, DC: American Psychiatric Press.

Hunt, D. J. (1989). Issues in working with Southeast Asian refugees. In *Crossing Cultures in Mental Health*, ed. D. R. Koslow and E. P. Salett, pp. 49–63. Washington, DC: SIETAR International.

Jacobson, E. (1954). The self and the object world. *Psychoanalytic Study of the Child* 9:75–127. New York: International Universities Press.

———— (1964). *The Self and the Object World*. New York: International Universities Press.

Janet, P. (1907). *The Major Symptoms of Hysteria*. New York: Macmillan.

Jenkins, L. (1994). African-American identity and its social context. In *Race, Ethnicity, and Self: Identity in Multicultural Perspective*, ed. E. P. Salett and D. R. Koslow, pp. 63–88. Washington, DC: National Multi-Cultural Institute.

Jones, E. (1928). Fear, guilt, and hate. In *Papers on Psychoanalysis*. Baltimore, MD: Williams & Wilkins, 1950.

Kafka, F. (1926). *The Castle*, trans. W. Muir and E. Muir. New York: Vintage, 1958.

Kagan, J. (1981). *The Second Year*. Cambridge, MA: Harvard University Press.

Kahn, C. (1997a). Conclusion. In *Immigrant Experiences: Personal Narrative and Psychological Analysis*, ed. P. H. Elovitz and C. Kahn, pp. 274–280. Cranbury, NJ: Associated University Presses.

———— (1997b). Four women: immigrants in cross-cultural marriages. In *Immigrant Experiences: Personal Narrative and Psychological Analysis*, ed. P. H. Elovitz and C. Kahn, pp. 199–220. Cranbury, NJ: Associated University Presses.

———— (1997c). Emigration without leaving home. In *Immigrant Experi-*

ences: Personal Narrative and Psychological Analysis, ed. P. H. Elovitz and C. Kahn, pp. 255–273. Cranbury, NJ: Associated University Presses.

Kakar, S. (1985). Psychoanalysis and non-western cultures *International Review of Psycho-Analysis* 12:441–448.

Kareem, J. (1992). The Nafsiyat Intercultural Therapy Centre: ideas and experience in intercultural therapy. In *Intercultural Therapy: Themes, Interpretations and Practice,* ed. J. Kareem and R. Littlewood, pp. 14–37. London: Blackwell Scientific Publications.

Kareem, J., and Littlewood, R., eds. (1992). *Intercultural Therapy: Themes, Interpretations and Practice.* London: Blackwell Scientific Publications.

Karpf, E. (1935). The choice of language in polyglot psychoanalysis. *Psychoanalytic Quarterly* 24:343–357.

Kernberg, O. F. (1967). Borderline personality organization. *Journal of the American Psychoanalytic Association* 15:641–685.

——— (1970). A psychoanalytic classification of character pathology. *Journal of the American Psychoanalytic Association* 18:800–822.

——— (1975). *Borderline Conditions and Pathological Narcissism.* New York: Jason Aronson.

——— (1976). *Object Relations Theory and Clinical Psychoanalysis.* New York: Jason Aronson.

——— (1980). *Internal World and External Reality.* New York: Jason Aronson.

——— (1984). *Severe Personality Disorders.* New Haven, CT: Yale University Press.

——— (1995). *Love Relations: Normality and Pathology.* New Haven, CT: Yale University Press.

Khan, M. (1974). *The Privacy of the Self.* New York: International Universities Press.

——— (1983). *Hidden Selves.* New York: International Universities Press.

Killingmo, B. (1989). Conflict and deficit: implications for technique. *International Journal of Psycho-Analysis* 70:65–79.

Klein, M. (1935). A contribution to the psychogenesis of manic-depressive states. In *Love, Guilt and Reparation and Other Works 1921–1945,* pp. 262–289. New York: Free Press, 1975.

——— (1937). Love, guilt and reparation. In *Love, Guilt and Reparation and Other Works 1921–1945.* New York: Free Press, 1975.

——— (1948). *Contributions to Psychoanalysis (1921–1945).* London: Hogarth.

Knafo, D., and Yaari, A. (1997). Leaving the promised land: Israeli immigrants in the United States. In *Immigrant Experiences: Personal Narrative and Psychological Analysis*, ed. P. H. Elovitz and C. Kahn, pp. 221–240. Cranbury, NJ: Associated University Presses.

Kohut, H. (1977). *Restoration of the Self.* New York: International Universities Press.

Kraepelin E. (1905). *Einfuehrung in die Psychiatrische Klinik*, 2nd ed. Leipzig, Germany: Barth.

Kraft-Goin, M. (1999). Transcultural psychiatry: overcoming the boundaries of culture. *Journal of Practical Psychiatry and Behavioral Health* 5: 56–58.

Kramer, S. (1980). Residues of split-object and split-self dichotomies in adolescence. In *Rapprochement: The Critical Subphase of Separation-Individuation*, ed. R. Lax, S. Bach, and J. A. Burland, pp. 417–437. New York: Jason Aronson.

Kristeva, J. (1988). *Étrangers à nous mêmes.* Paris: Fayard.

Krystal, H. (1966). Giorgio de Chirico: ego states and artistic production. *American Imago* 23:210–226.

Krystal, H., and Petty, T. A. (1963). Dynamics of adjustment to migration. In *Proceedings of the III World Congress of Psychiatry and Psychiatric Quarterly Supplement*, 37:118–133.

Kurtz, S. A. (1988). The psychoanalysis of time. *Journal of the American Psychoanalytic Association* 36:985–1094.

Lacayo, R. (1984). Meeting of two masters: Sir David Lean and Lord Snowdon take aim at *A Passage to India. Time*, August 27, pp. 54–55.

Lagache, D. (1956). Sur le polyglottisme dans l'analyse. *La Psychoanalyse* 1:167–178.

Lager, E., and Zwerling, I. (1980). Time orientation and psychotherapy in the ghetto. *American Journal of Psychiatry* 137:306–309.

Lapierre, D. (1985). *City of Joy.* New York: Doubleday.

Leary, K. (1995). Interpreting in the dark: race and ethnicity in psychoanalytic psychotherapy. *Psychoanalytic Psychology* 12:127–140.

——— (1997). Race, self-disclosure, and "forbidden talk": race and ethnicity in contemporary clinical practice. *Psychoanalytic Quarterly* 66:163–189.

Levinson, D. J., Darrow, C. M., Klein, E. B., et al. (1978). *The Seasons of a Man's Life.* New York: Knopf.

Lewin, R. A., and Schulz, C. (1992). *Losing and Fusing: Borderline Transitional Object and Self Relations.* Northvale, NJ: Jason Aronson.

Lewis, M., and Brooks-Gunn J. (1979). *Social Cognition and the Acquisition of Self.* New York: Plenum.

Lichtenstein, H. (1961). Identity and sexuality: a study of their inter-relationship in man. *Journal of the American Psychoanalytic Association* 9:179–260.

———— (1963). The dilemma of human identity: notes on self-transformation, self-objectivation and metamorphosis. *Journal of the American Psychoanalytic Association* 11:173–223.

Limentani, A. (1989). *Between Freud and Klein: The Psychoanalytic Quest for Knowledge and Truth.* London: Free Association.

Littlewood, R. (1992a). Towards an intercultural therapy. In *Intercultural Therapy: Themes, Interpretations and Practice,* ed. J. Kareem and R. Littlewood, pp. 3–13. London: Blackwell Scientific Publications.

———— (1992b). How universal is something we can call "therapy"? In *Intercultural Therapy: Themes, Interpretations and Practice,* ed. J. Kareem and R. Littlewood, pp. 38–56. London: Blackwell Scientific Publications.

Littlewood, R., and Lipsedge, M. (1989). *Aliens and Alienists: Ethnic Minorities and Psychiatry.* London: Unwin Hyman.

Loewald, H. W. (1951). Ego and reality. *International Journal of Psycho-Analysis* 32:10–21.

———— (1960). On the therapeutic action of psychoanalysis. *International Journal of Psycho-Analysis* 41:16–33.

Madow, L. (1997). On the way to a second symbiosis. In *The Seasons of Life: Separation-Individuation Perspectives,* ed. S. Akhtar and S. Kramer, pp. 157–170. Northvale, NJ: Jason Aronson.

Mahler, M. S. (1958a). Autism and symbiosis: two extreme disturbances of identity. *International Journal of Psycho-Analysis* 39:77–83.

———— (1958b). On two crucial phases of integration of the sense of identity: separation-individuation and bisexual identity. *Journal of the American Psychoanalytic Association* 6:136–139.

———— (1967). On human symbiosis and the vicissitudes of individuation. In *The Selected Papers of Margaret S. Mahler,* vol. 2, pp. 77–98. New York: Jason Aronson.

———— (1972). A study of the separation and individuation process and its possible application to borderline phenomena in the psychoanalytic situation. *Psychoanalytic Study of the Child* 26:403–424. New Haven, CT: Yale University Press.

———— (1974). Symbiosis and individuation: the psychological birth of the human infant. In *The Selected Papers of Margaret S. Mahler,* vol. 2, pp. 149–165. New York: Jason Aronson, 1979.

Mahler, M. S., and Furer, M. (1968). *On Human Symbiosis and the Vicissitudes of Individuation*. New York: International Universities Press.

Mahler, M. S., and Gosliner, B. J. (1955). On symbiotic child psychosis: genetic, dynamic, and restitutive aspects. *Psychoanalytic Study of the Child* 10:195–212. New York: International Universities Press.

Mahler, M. S., Pine, F., and Bergman, A. (1975). *The Psychological Birth of the Human Infant*. New York: Basic Books.

Manalansan, M. (1996). Searching for community: Filipino gay men in New York City. In *Asian American Sexualities: Dimensions of the Gay and Lesbian Experience*, ed. R. C. Leong, pp. 83–101. New York: Routledge.

Marlin, O. (1997). Fleeing toward the new and yearning for the old. In *Immigrant Experiences: Personal Narrative and Psychological Analysis*, ed. P. H. Elovitz and C. Kahn, pp. 241–254. Cranbury, NJ: Associated University Presses.

Martinez, I. Z. (1994). Quien soy? Who am I? Identity issues for Puerto Rican adolescents. In *Race, Ethnicity, and Self: Identity in Multicultural Perspective*, ed. E. P. Salett and D. R. Koslow, pp. 89–116. Washington, DC: National Multi-Cultural Institute.

Maslow, A. (1971). *The Farther Reaches of Human Nature*. New York: Viking.

Masson, J. M. (1985). *The Complete Letters of Sigmund Freud to Wilhelm Fliess*. Cambridge, MA: Harvard University Press.

Masterson J. F. (1976). *Psychotherapy of the Borderline Adult: A Developmental Approach*. New York: Brunner/Mazel.

Meaders, N. Y. (1997). The transcultural self. In *Immigrant Experiences: Personal Narrative and Psychological Analysis*, ed. P. H. Elovitz and C. Kahn, pp. 47–59. Cranbury, NJ: Associated University Presses.

Mehta, P. (1995). Michigan analysts engage the Indo-Pakistani community. *American Psychoanalyst* 29:2, 6–7.

——— (1997). The import and export of psychoanalysis: India. *Journal of the American Academy of Psychoanalysis* 25:455–472.

——— (1998). The emergence, conflicts, and integration of the bicultural self: psychoanalysis of an adolescent daughter of South-Asian immigrant parents. In *The Colors of Childhood: Separation-Individuation Across Cultural, Racial, and Ethnic Differences*, ed. S. Akhtar and S. Kramer, pp. 129–168. Northvale, NJ: Jason Aronson.

Menges, L. J. (1959). *Adequacy for Migrating: An Investigation of Some Psychological Aspects of Migration*. The Hague: University of Leiden Press.

Merriam-Webster's Ninth New Collegiate Dictionary. (1987). Springfield, MA: Merriam-Webster Inc.

Mistral, G. (1971). *Selected Poems of Gabriela Mistral,* trans. and ed. D. Dana. Baltimore, MD: Johns Hopkins University Press.

Modell, A. (1965). On aspects of the superego's development. *International Journal of Psycho-Analysis* 46:323–331.

——— (1976). The holding environment and the therapeutic action of psychoanalysis. *Journal of the American Psychoanalytic Association* 24:285–307.

——— (1984). *Psychoanalysis in a New Context.* New York: International Universities Press.

Mollica, R. F. (1989). Developing effective mental health policies and services for traumatized refugee patients. In *Crossing Cultures in Mental Health,* ed. D. R. Koslow and E. P. Salett, pp. 101–115. Washington, DC: SIETAR International.

Money J., and Ehrhardt, A. (1972). *Man, Woman, Boy and Girl.* Baltimore: Johns Hopkins University Press.

Moore, B., and Fine, B. (1990). *Psychoanalytic Terms and Concepts.* New York: American Psychoanalytic Association.

Morley, J. D. (1985). *Pictures from the Water Trade.* Boston: Atlantic Monthly Press.

Moskowitz, M. (1996). The social conscience of psychoanalysis. In *Reaching Across Boundaries of Culture and Class,* ed. R. Pérez Foster, M. Moskowitz, and R. A. Javier, pp. 21–46. Northvale, NJ: Jason Aronson.

Mura, D. (1991). *Turning Japanese: Memoirs of a Sansei.* New York: Atlantic Monthly Press.

Neki, J. S. (1975). Psychotherapy in India: past, present, and future. *American Journal of Psychotherapy* 79:92–100.

Ng, M. L. (1985). Psychoanalysis for the Chinese: applicable or not applicable? *International Review of Psycho-Analysis* 12:449–460.

Niederland, W. (1968). Clinical observations on the "Survivor Syndrome." *International Journal of Psycho-Analysis* 49:313–315.

Obendorf, C. P. (1950). Unsatisfactory results of psychoanalytic therapy. *Psychoanalytic Quarterly* 19:393–407.

Ogden, T. (1995). *Subjects of Analysis.* Northvale, NJ: Jason Aronson.

Olesker, W. (1990). Sex differences during the early separation-individuation process: implications for gender identity formation. *Journal of the American Psychoanalytic Association* 38:325–346.

Oremland, J. D. (1973). Specific dreams during the termination phase. *Journal of the American Psychoanalytic Association* 21:285–302.

Pande, S. K. (1968). The mystique of "Western" psychotherapy": an Eastern interpretation. *Journal of Nervous and Mental Disease* 146:425–432.

Parens, H. (1998). The impact of cultural holding environment on psychic development. In *The Colors of Childhood: Separation-Individuation Across Cultural, Racial, and Ethnic Differences*, ed. S. Akhtar and S. Kramer, pp. 199–230. Northvale, NJ: Jason Aronson.

Pérez Foster, R. (1996). Assessing the psychodynamic function of language in the bilingual patient. In *Reaching Across Boundaries of Culture and Class*, ed. R. Pérez Foster, M. Moskowitz, and R. A. Javier, p. 243–263. Northvale, NJ: Jason Aronson.

Pérez Foster, R., Moskowitz, M., and Javier, R. A., eds. (1996). *Reaching Across Boundaries of Culture and Class*. Northvale, NJ: Jason Aronson.

Pfeiffer, E. (1974). Borderline states. *Diseases of the Nervous System* 35:212–219.

Phinney, J. S., Lochner, B. T., and Murphy, R. (1990). Ethnic identity development and psychological adjustment in adolescence. In *Ethnic Issues in Adolescent Mental Health*, ed. A. R. Stiffman and L. E. Davis, pp. 53–73. Newbury Park, CA: Sage.

Pine, F. (1997). *Diversity and Direction in Psychoanalytic Technique*. New Haven, CT: Yale University Press.

Piontelli, A. (1987). Infant observation from before birth. *International Journal of Psycho-Analysis* 68:453–463.

———— (1988). Pre-natal life, reflected in the analysis of a psychotic girl at age two. *International Review of Psycho-Analysis* 15:73–81.

Poland, W. (1975). Tact as a psychoanalytic function. *International Journal of Psycho-Analysis* 56:155–161.

Pollock, G. (1989). On migration—voluntary and coerced. *The Annual of Psychoanalysis* 17:145–169.

Poznanski, E. O. (1972). The "replacement child": a saga of unresolved parental grief. *Behavioral Pediatrics* 81:1190–1193.

Prathikanti, S. (1997). East Indian American families. In *Working with Asian Americans: A Guide for Clinicians*, ed. E. Lee, pp. 79–100. New York: Guilford.

Prince, M. (1905). *The Dissociation of a Personality*. New York: Longmans.

Pulver, S. (1993). The eclectic analyst, or the many roads to insight and change. *Journal of the American Psychoanalytic Association* 41:339–357.

Ramanajum, B. K. (1997). The process of acculturation among Asian-Indian immigrants. In *Immigrant Experiences: Personal Narrative and Psychological Analysis*, ed. P. H. Elovitz and C. Kahn, pp. 139–147. Cranbury, NJ: Associated University Presses.

Rapaport, D. (1960). The structure of psychoanalytic theory. *Psychological Issues* 6:39–72.

Rendon, M. (1996). Psychoanalysis in historic-economic perspective. In *Reaching Across Boundaries of Culture and Class*, ed. R. Pérez Foster, M. Moskowitz, and R. A. Javier, pp. 47–70. Northvale, NJ: Jason Aronson.

Rinsley, D. B. (1982). *Borderline and Other Self Disorders: A Developmental and Object Relations Perspective.* New York: Jason Aronson.

Ritsner, M., Mirsky, J., Factourovich, A., et al. (1993). Psychological adjustment and distress among Soviet immigrant physicians: demographic and background variables. *Israel Journal of Psychiatry* 30:244–254.

Roheim, G. (1943). *The Origin and Function of Culture.* New York: International Universities Press.

———— (1952). *The Gates of the Dream.* New York: International Universities Press.

Roland, A. (1988). *In Search of Self in India and Japan: Toward a Cross-Cultural Psychology.* Princeton, NJ: Princeton University Press.

———— (1996). *Cultural Pluralism and Psychoanalysis: The Asian and North American Experience.* New York: Routledge.

———— (1997). Indians in America: adaptation and the bicultural self. In *Immigrant Experiences: Personal Narrative and Psychological Analysis*, ed. P. H. Elovitz and C. Kahn, pp. 148–157. Cranbury, NJ: Associated University Presses.

Rosenfeld, H. (1987). The influence of projective identification in the analyst's task. In *Impasse and Interpretation*, pp. 157–261. London: Tavistock.

Ross, J. M. (1979). Fathering: a review of some psychoanalytic contributions on paternity. *International Journal of Psycho-Analysis* 60:317–327.

———— (1982). Oedipus revisited: Laius and the Laius complex. *Psychoanalytic Study of the Child* 37:169–192. New Haven, CT: Yale University Press.

———— (1990). The eye of the beholder: on the developmental dialogue between fathers and daughters. In *New Dimensions in Adult Development*, ed. R. A. Nemiroff and C. A. Colarusso, pp. 47–72. New York: Basic Books.

———— (1994). *What Men Want.* Cambridge, MA: Harvard University Press.

———— (1996). Male infidelity in long marriages: second adolescences and fourth individuations. In *Intimacy and Infidelity: Separation-Individuation Perspectives*, ed. S. Akhtar and S. Kramer, pp. 107–130. Northvale, NJ: Jason Aronson.

Rushdie, S. (1980). *Midnight's Children.* New York: Knopf.

———— (1989). *Satanic Verses.* New York: Viking.

Saavedra, C. C. (1986). Unemployed. In *Anthology of Contemporary Latin American Literature 1960–1984*, ed. B. J. Luby and W. H. Finke, p. 94. Cranbury, NJ: Associated University Presses.

Sabelli, H. C. (1997). Becoming Hispanic, becoming American: Latin American immigrants' journey to national identity. In *Immigrant Experiences: Personal Narrative and Psychological Analysis*, ed. P. H. Elovitz and C. Kahn, pp. 158–179. Cranbury, NJ: Associated University Presses.

Sack, W., Angell, R., Kinzie, J. D., et al. (1986). Psychiatric effects of massive trauma on Cambodian children: II: the family and the school. *Journal of the American Academy of Child Psychiatrists* 25:377–383.

Santini, I. (1999). Mutuality and concern: evolving social affiliation. Proceedings of the IPA-UNESCO Congress: At the Threshold of the Millennium, Lima, Peru, April 1998 (in press).

Schachter, J., Martin, G. C., Gundle, M. J., and O'Neil, M. K. (1997). Clinical experience with psychoanalytic post-termination meetings. *International Journal of Psycho-Analysis* 78:1183–1198.

Schilder, P. (1935). *The Image and Appearance of the Human Body*. New York: International Universities Press.

Schlessinger, N., and Robbins, F. P. (1983). *A Developmental View of the Psychoanalytic Process*. New York: International Universities Press.

Schreuder, B. J. N. (1999). *The transitional space between inner and outer world in migration and psychodrama*. Presented at the Symposium "Migrants and Refugees: About Mourning, Coping, and Identity," co-sponsored by the Dutch Psychoanalytic Society and PHAROS (The Dutch Mental Health Organization for Migrants and Refugees), Amsterdam, March.

Searles, H. F. (1960). *The Non-Human Environment in Normal Development and Schizophrenia*. New York: International Universities Press.

——— (1977). Dual- and multiple-identity processes in borderline ego functioning. In *Borderline Personality Disorders: The Concept, the Syndrome, the Patient*. New York: International Universities Press.

——— (1986). *My Work with Borderline Patients*. Northvale, NJ: Jason Aronson.

Settlage, C. F. (1991). On the treatment of preoedipal pathology. In *Beyond the Symbiotic Orbit: Advances in Separation-Individuation Theory—Essays in Honor of Selma Kramer, M.D.*, ed. S. Akhtar and H. Parens, pp. 351–367. Hillsdale, NJ: Analytic Press.

——— (1992). Psychoanalytic observations on adult development in life and in the therapeutic relationship. *Psychoanalysis and Contemporary Thought* 15:349–374.

———— (1993). Therapeutic process in the restructuring of object and self constancy. *Journal of the American Psychoanalytic Association* 41:473–492.

———— (1994). On the contribution of separation-individuation theory to psychoanalysis: developmental process, pathogenesis, therapeutic process, and technique. In *Mahler and Kohut: Perspectives on Development, Psychopathology, and Technique,* ed. S. Kramer and S. Akhtar, pp. 17–52. Northvale, NJ: Jason Aronson.

Shapiro, E. T., and Pinsker, H. (1973). Shared ethnic scotoma. *American Journal of Psychiatry* 130:1338–1341.

Shengold, L. (1989). *Soul Murder: The Effects of Childhood Abuse and Deprivation.* New Haven, CT: Yale University Press.

Shokeid, M. (1988). *Children of Circumstance: Israeli Emigrants in New York.* Ithaca, NY: Cornell University Press.

Silber, N. (1994). *The Romance of Reunion: Northerners and the South, 1865–1900.* Chapel Hill, NC: University of North Carolina Press.

Slater, E., and Roth, M. (1969). *Clinical Psychiatry,* 34th ed. Baltimore: Williams & Wilkins.

Smolar, A. (1999). Bridging the gap: technical aspects of the analysis of a narcissistic immigrant. *Journal of Clinical Psychoanalysis* (in press).

Solzhenitsyn, A. (1969). *Cancer Ward,* Part I, Chapter 14. New York: Farrar, Straus and Giroux.

Stengel, E. (1939). On learning a new language. *International Journal of Psycho-Analysis* 20:471–479.

Stepansky, P. E. (1988). *The Memoirs of Margaret S. Mahler.* New York: Free Press.

Sterba, E. (1934). Homesickness and the mother's breast. *Psychiatric Quarterly* 14:701–707.

Stern, D. N. (1985). *The Interpersonal World of the Infant.* New York: Basic Books.

Stoller, R. (1968). *Sex and Gender.* New York: Science House.

Stolorow, R. D., and Atwood, G. E. (1989). Unconscious fantasy: an intersubjective-developmental perspective. *Psychoanalytic Inquiry* 9:364–369.

Strachey, J. (1934). The nature of the therapeutic action of psychoanalysis. *International Journal of Psycho-Analysis* 15:157–159.

Strachey, J., Freud, A., Strachey, A., and Tyson, A. (1923). Editor's introduction, pp. 3–11. In *The Ego and the Id,* Freud, S. *Standard Edition* 19: 1–66.

Strenger, C. (1989). The classic and romantic visions in psychoanalysis. *International Journal of Psycho-Analysis* 70:595–610.

Surya, N. C., and Jayaram, S. S. (1964). Some basic considerations of psychotherapy in India. *Indian Journal of Psychiatry* 3:153–156.

Taketomo, Y. (1989). An American-Japanese transcultural psychoanalysis and the issue of teacher transference. *Journal of the American Academy of Psychoanalysis* 17:427–450.

Tang, N. M. (1992). Some psychoanalytic implications of Chinese philosophy and child-rearing practices. *Psychoanalytic Study of the Child* 47:371–389. New Haven, CT: International Universities Press.

Tang, N. M., and Gardner, J. (1999). Race, culture, and psychotherapy: transference to minority therapists. *Psychoanalytic Quarterly* 68:1–20.

Tausk, V. (1919). Uber die enstehung des beeinflussungsapparates in der schizophrenie. *International Journal of Psycho-Analysis* 5:1–33.

Taylor, O. L. (1989). The effects of cultural assumptions on cross-cultural communication. In *Crossing Cultures in Mental Health*, ed. D. R. Koslow and E. P. Salett, pp. 18–30. Washington, DC: SIETAR International.

Teja, J. S., and Akhtar, S. (1981). The psycho-social problems of FMG's with special references to those in psychiatry. In *Foreign Medical Graduates in Psychiatry: Issues and Problems*, ed. R. S. Chen, pp. 321–338. New York: Human Sciences Press.

Thomas, A., and Chess, S. (1977). *Temperament and Development.* New York: Brunner/Mazel.

——— (1984). Genesis and evolution of behavioral disorders: from infancy to early adult life. *American Journal of Psychiatry* 141:1–9.

Thomson, J. A., Harris, M., and Volkan, V. (1993). *The Psychology of Western European Neo-Racism.* Charlottesville, VA: Center for the Study of Mind and Human Interaction.

Ticho, G. (1971). Cultural aspects of transference and countertransference. *Bulletin of the Menninger Clinic* 35:313–326.

Trilling, L. (1968). *From Sincerity to Authenticity.* Cambridge, MA: Harvard University Press.

Tummala, P. (1998). Review of *Working with Asian Americans: A Guide for Clinicians*, ed. E. Lee. *American Family Therapy Academy Newsletter* 73: 32–34.

Vallejo, C. (1923). No one lives in the house anymore. In *The Complete Posthumous Poetry*, trans. C. Eshleman and J. R. Garcia, p. 27. Berkeley: University of California Press, 1980.

Van Essen, J. (1999). Of fatherland and motherland: love and hate in adolescent refugees. In *Proceedings of the IPA–UNESCO Congress: At the Threshold of the Millennium*, Lima, Peru, April 1998 (in press).

Van Waning, A. (1999). Time collapse and fragmentation: the haunting past in the life of a refugee. In *Proceedings of the IPA–UNESCO Congress: At the Threshold of the Millennium*, Lima, Peru, April 1998 (in press).

Volkan, V. D. (1976). *Primitive Internalized Object Relations*. New York: International Universities Press.

—— (1981). *Linking Objects and Linking Phenomena: A Study of the Form, Symptoms, Metapsychology and Therapy of Complicated Mourning*. New York: International Universities Press.

—— (1987). *Six Steps in the Treatment of Borderline Personality Organization*. Northvale, NJ: Jason Aronson.

—— (1988). *The Need to Have Enemies and Allies*. Northvale, NJ: Jason Aronson.

—— (1990). Review of *Psychoanalytic Perspectives on Migration and Exile*, by L. Grinberg and R. Grinberg. *International Journal of Psycho-Analysis* 71:541–543.

—— (1993). Immigrants and refugees: a psychodynamic perspective. *Mind and Human Interaction* 4:63–69.

—— (1997). *Blood Lines: From Ethnic Price to Ethnic Terrorism*. New York: Farrar, Straus and Giroux.

—— (1999). Nostalgia as a linking phenomenon. *Journal of Applied Psychoanalytic Studies* 1(2):169–179.

Volkan, V. D., and Corney, R. T. (1968). Some considerations of satellite states and satellite dreams. *British Journal of Medical Psychology* 41:283–290.

Waelder, R. (1936). The principle of multiple function: observations on multiple determination. *Psychoanalytic Quarterly* 5:45–62.

Wallerstein, R. S. (1990). Psychoanalysis: the common ground. *International Journal of Psycho-Analysis* 71:3–20.

Wangh, M. (1992). Being a refugee and being an immigrant. *International Psychoanalysis*, winter:15–17.

Ward, I. (1993). Examining Freud's "phantasy" about England. *Psychiatric Times* 10:38.

Weil, A. (1970). The basic core. *Psychoanalytic Study of the Child* 25:442–460. New York: International Unniversities Press.

Werman, D. S. (1977). Normal and pathological nostalgia. *Journal of the American Psychoanalytic Association* 25:387–398.

Westermeyer, J. (1990). Motivations for uprooting and migration. In *Mental Health of Immigrants and Refugees*, ed. W. H. Holtzman and T. H. Bornemann, pp. 78–89. Austin, TX: University of Texas Press.

Wheelis, A. (1958). *The Quest for Identity*. New York: Norton.

Winnicott, D. W. (1935). The manic defense. In *Through Paediatrics to Psycho-Analysis*, pp. 129–144. New York: Brunner/Mazel, 1992.

——— (1949). Mind and its relation to the psyche-soma. In *Through Paediatrics to Psychoanalysis*, pp. 243–255. New York: Brunner/Mazel, 1953.

——— (1953). Transitional objects and transitional phenomena. In *Through Paediatrics to Psycho-Analysis*, pp. 229–242. New York: Brunner/Mazel.

——— (1960a). The theory of parent–infant relationship. In *The Maturational Processes and the Facilitating Environment*, pp. 37–55. New York: International Universities Press, 1965.

——— (1960b). Ego distortion in terms of true and false self. In *The Maturational Processes and the Facilitating Environment*, pp. 140–152. New York: International Universities Press, 1965.

——— (1963). The development of the capacity for concern. In *The Maturational Processes and the Facilitating Environment*, pp. 73–82. New York: International Universities Press, 1965.

——— (1971). *Playing and Reality*. London: Tavistock.

Wolf, E. (1994). Selfobject experiences: development, psychopathology, treatment. In *Mahler and Kohut: Perspectives on Development, Psychopathology and Treatment*, ed. S. Kramer and S. Akhtar, pp. 65–96. Northvale, NJ: Jason Aronson.

Wolman, T., and Thompson, T. L. T. (1990). Adult development. In *Human Behavior: An Introduction for Medical Students*, ed. A. Stoudemire, pp. 178–205. Philadelphia: Lippincott.

Yamamoto, J., and Wagatsuma, H. (1980). The Japanese and Japanese American. *Journal of Operational Psychiatry* 11:120–135.

Zafar, B. S. (1862). *Inkikhab-e-Zafar*, p. 89. New Delhi: Maktaba Jamia, 1971.

Zaphiropoulos, M. L. (1982). Transcultural parameters in the transference and countertransference. *Journal of the American Academy of Psychoanalysis* 10:571–584.

Zerubavel, E. (1991). *The Fine Line: Making Distinctions in Everyday Life*. New York: Free Press.

CREDITS

Small segments of Chapters 1 and 4 and somewhat larger portions of Chapter 3 are reprinted from "A Third Individuation: Immigration, Identity, and the Psychoanalytic Process," *Journal of the American Psychoanalytic Association* 43(4):1051–1084, 1995, with the permission of International Universities Press, Madison, CT. Portions of Chapter 2 have appeared in "The Concept of Identity: Developmental Origins, Phenomenology, Clinical Relevance, and Measurement," *Harvard Review of Psychiatry* 3:254–267, 1996, and are reprinted with the permission of co-author Steve Samuel, Ph.D., and the Oxford University Press.

The extract from Luo Fu's poem "Outside the Window" is reprinted from *Anthology of Modern Chinese Poetry* (ed. and transl. M. Yeh) with the permission of Yale University Press © 1992. The extracts from Indran Amrithanayagam's poem "What Happened to All My Life," Darius Cooper's poem "I have Been Offered My Country's Begging Bowl Again," and Reinzi Crusz's poem "Conversations with God about My Present Whereabouts," are reprinted from *Living in America: Poetry and Fiction by South Asian American Writers* (ed. R. Rustonji-Kearns) with the permission of Westview Press © 1995. Lines from the poem by J. Brodsky are used with the permission of Farrar, Straus, and Giroux. The author expresses his gratitude to those whose names appear above for permission to use the passages indicated. Every effort has been made to ascertain the owner of copyrights for the selections used in this volume and to obtain permission to reprint copyrighted passages. The author will be pleased, in subsequent editions, to correct any inadvertent error or omission that may be pointed out.

INDEX

ABOUT THE AUTHOR

Salman Akhtar, M.D., is Professor of Psychiatry at Jefferson Medical College, Lecturer on Psychiatry at Harvard Medical School, and Training and Supervising Analyst at the Philadelphia Psychoanalytic Institute. He is the Book Review Editor of the *Journal of Applied Psychoanalytic Studies,* an associate editor of the *Journal of Psychotherapy Practice and Research,* member of the editorial board of the *Journal of the American Psychoanalytic Association,* past member of the editorial board of the *International Journal of Psycho-Analysis,* and an editorial reader for *Psychoanalytic Quarterly.* He is the author of *Broken Structures: Severe Personality Disorders and Their Treatment* (1992), *Quest for Answers: A Primer for Understanding and Treating Severe Personality Disorders* (1995), and *Inner Torment* (1999). His more than 140 scientific publications also include fifteen edited or co-edited books. Dr. Akhtar is the recipient of the Journal of the American Psychoanalytic Association's Award (1995) and the Margaret Mahler Literature Prize (1996), and was named the 1998 Clinician of the Year by IPTAR, New York. He has also published five volumes of poetry.